Geraldo Bezerra da Silva Junior
Maria Cecília C. Barreira

Educational technology for people with chronic kidney disease

Geraldo Bezerra da Silva Junior
Maria Cecília C. Barreira

Educational technology for people with chronic kidney disease

Construction and validation process

Imprint

Any brand names and product names mentioned in this book are subject to trademark, brand or patent protection and are trademarks or registered trademarks of their respective holders. The use of brand names, product names, common names, trade names, product descriptions etc. even without a particular marking in this work is in no way to be construed to mean that such names may be regarded as unrestricted in respect of trademark and brand protection legislation and could thus be used by anyone.

Cover image: www.ingimage.com

This book is a translation from the original published under ISBN 978-613-9-63649-5.

Publisher:
Sciencia Scripts
is a trademark of
Dodo Books Indian Ocean Ltd. and OmniScriptum S.R.L publishing group

120 High Road, East Finchley, London, N2 9ED, United Kingdom
Str. Armeneasca 28/1, office 1, Chisinau MD-2012, Republic of Moldova, Europe
Printed at: see last page
ISBN: 978-620-7-69304-7

DEDICATORY

To *my parents, who have always encouraged me and spared no effort to offer me opportunities for personal and professional growth, and for all the love they have shown me.*

To you, with much love.

ACKNOWLEDGEMENTS

Firstly, I would like to thank God for guiding me and giving me the wisdom to face everyday obstacles and not give up on pursuing my dreams, always showing me the way.

To my parents, Hélio and Cacilda, who, ever since I was a child, showed me the importance of studying and, at times, sacrificed their lives to give me the opportunity to study at institutions that would bring me growth. Thank you for all your love, complicity and support.

To my husband, a partner of ten and an encourager of a thousand. He was always there cheering me on, from the moment I was selected for my master's degree, and he accompanied me through nights of lost sleep, moments of anxiety, worry and fear, always with an outstretched hand and a "you can do it" that gave me the strength to keep going.

To my sister, Bel, and all the family and friends who had the patience and understanding to be told "I can't" in response to many invitations to go out.

To my advisor, Prof Dr Geraldo Bezerra da Silva Júnior, for his availability, for all the knowledge he shared, for the injections of encouragement I received whenever I met him and for everything he added to me as a person and as a professional. I always say that he is an angel in my life.

I would like to thank Prof Dr Zélia Maria de Sousa Araújo Santos, whom I have become a fan of, not only for her enormous baggage of scientific knowledge, but also for the peace of mind she conveys and her willingness to always help me.

To all the professionals who kindly agreed to take part in the research and collaborate in carrying out this work.

To the members of the board, Prof Dr Zélia Maria de Souza Araújo Santos, Prof Dr Danielle Teixeira Queiroz, Prof Dr Edson Lopes da Ponte and Prof Dr Ana Maria Fontenelle Catrib, for their willingness to help enrich and improve this work.

To the staff of the master's programme who were always willing to help.

To my bosses, who helped me in many ways to fulfil the difficult task of dedicating myself to my master's degree and working at the same time. Thank you for your patience, understanding and encouragement.

To all those who contributed in some way to the realisation of this work.

Thank you so much!

SUMMARY

Chronic kidney disease (CKD) is a syndrome of progressive and irreversible loss of kidney function, the main causes of which are systemic arterial hypertension (SAH), diabetes mellitus (DM) and chronic glomerulonephritis. Education and health promotion activities carried out in groups can help raise the level of knowledge, acceptance of their limits and awareness of positive attitudes. Educational work with groups is an important alternative for Educational Technology in Health, with the aim of promoting health and deepening discussions and knowledge, enabling people to improve their level of autonomy and, consequently, their quality of life. This is a descriptive methodological study to build and validate an educational technology and tool for recording information related to the treatment of CKD. The study was carried out in Dialysis Clinics located in the city of Fortaleza, capital of Ceará, with the participation of doctors and nurses who had been working in these centres for at least 2 years. The professionals consulted evaluated the Educational Technology Proposal using a questionnaire based on feasibility and applicability. The data from this instrument showed that 9 (75%) considered the technology to be feasible. According to 8 of the participants (66.6%), the ETP addresses preventive behaviours for CKD. For the majority of participants (75%), the TPP makes an important contribution to the work of professionals in preventing complications resulting from CKD. Most of the participants (83.3%) reported that TEP was very important for people with CKD in terms of changing their habits, adapting to treatment and improving their quality of life. It was even suggested that the project be extended to outpatient clinics (to include people on conservative treatment) and not be restricted to dialysis centres. A number of suggestions were made by the professionals and were taken into account in the construction of the tool for monitoring people with CKD. The aim of creating this tool was to better record the information related to the treatment of people with CKD and to enable better monitoring of the individual at all appointments, making it easier for the whole team to get to know their state of health and enabling them to be identified as having a chronic illness that requires special care.

Keywords: Chronic renal failure. Disease Prevention. Educational Technology.

SUMMARY

CHAPTER 1

INTRODUCTION

In recent decades there has been a marked reduction in mortality due to infectious and parasitic causes in Brazil, as a result of specific health measures such as the control and eradication of major epidemics, basic sanitation, advances in antibiotic therapy, contributing to an increase in life expectancy and an ageing population. At the same time, the progressive increase in industrialisation and urbanisation has meant that chronic-degenerative diseases have taken on a prominent role in the population's health, in addition to changes in lifestyle habits (BARBOSA et al, 2006).

The Brazilian Ministry of Health cites chronic diseases as the main causes of death in the world, as they are associated with a high number of premature deaths, loss of quality of life and generate a major economic impact for society in general. Among the main risk factors are smoking, unhealthy eating, a sedentary lifestyle and alcohol consumption (BRASIL, 2011).

Through the plan to tackle chronic non-communicable diseases, the Ministry of Health has implemented important policies to tackle chronic diseases, especially the Organisation for the Surveillance of Chronic Non-Communicable Diseases (NCDs), the aim of which is to learn about the distribution, magnitude, trends, problems and risk factors of chronic diseases, as well as to support public health promotion policies.

Chronic non-communicable diseases (NCDs) are responsible for around 60 per cent of deaths worldwide, affecting around 35 million people a year. For the next decade, it is expected that there will be a 17 per cent increase in mortality caused by NCDs (BRASIL, 2014).

Chronic kidney disease (CKD) is a major public health problem worldwide. For some years now, the number of people requiring care programmes to control and treat CKD has been increasing significantly (QUEIROZ, 2008).

Lewis (2010) highlights CKD as a serious public health problem in the United States, with around 26 million people suffering from the disease in its various stages. The prevalence rate of CKD has risen by more than 100 per cent in 10 years and the trend continues to grow. In Japan, according to Nozaki (2005), the number of people on dialysis had already passed 200,000 in 2002.

The Brazilian Dialysis Census Report presented data from 2013 in Brazil (SESSO et *al.,* 2014). The total estimated number of CKD patients in the country on 1 July 2013 was 100,397. The number has been gradually increasing over the years: 97,586 in 2012, 91,314 in 2011, and 54,523 in

2003. Half of these individuals were in the Southeast. The estimated number of people starting treatment in 2013 in Brazil was 34,161, corresponding to an incidence rate of 170 people per million population (pmp). The estimated incidence rate in 2012 and 2011 was 177 and 149 people pmp, respectively.

Silva (2013) points out that mortality from CKD is high worldwide and the main causes are Systemic Arterial Hypertension (SAH) and Diabetes Mellitus (DM) in Brazil, reflecting the clinical situation of people when they start dialysis, associated with low access to secondary prevention in CKD.

Health costs for people on dialysis increase every year, but if primary care were more effective in controlling the main causes of CKD (SAH and DM), many cases would be avoided, costs would be reduced in the long term and the quality of life of these people could be improved (CLARKSON, 2010).

Early recognition of the disease and the degree of kidney dysfunction are of the utmost importance for directing treatment. In order for CKD to be detected early, an initial assessment is required, in which tests such as a urine summary (urine I) and an estimate of the glomerular filtration rate (Cockroft-Gault equations and the Modification of Diet in Renal Disease study) are requested, in addition to determining the duration of the disease (K/DOQI, 2002). Late diagnosis limits treatment options, leading people to haemodialysis or transplantation, causing negative impacts on the quality of life of individuals and generating high costs for the SUS (SILVA, 2013).

Rocha (2010) emphasises the technological and therapeutic advances in the field of dialysis as important for increasing the survival of CKD patients, but points out that these advances have not improved the quality of life of these individuals.

According to Clarkson (2010) many CKD sufferers, when they are informed of the need to dialyse, go through a moment of shock, as they and their families are suddenly thrown into a sudden change of lifestyle (due to the urgency) and confronted with countless challenges, with little or no preparation for the start of dialysis. Therefore, the method of inserting the individual into this new reality leaves a gap in terms of education.

A study by Gricio, Kusumota and Cândido (2009) concluded that the majority of CKD patients undergoing conservative treatment have insufficient information about the disease and treatment modalities (including dialysis and transplantation), which can be a negative factor in adherence to treatment and can result in poor control of the disease and its complications.

It is extremely important to advise CKD sufferers about the disease itself, the treatment, the forms of renal replacement therapy and the risks and benefits of each of them, the needs and care related to vascular access (arterio-venous fistula or peritoneal dialysis catheter), dietary care (including the need to restrict water and certain foods), the use of medication (including the need to avoid nephrotoxic drugs), blood pressure and glycaemic control (ROCHA, 2010). This highlights the complexity of treatment and measures to prevent complications in CKD and the need for multidisciplinary team monitoring, which requires ongoing guidance (health education) for these people.

Lewis (2010) emphasises the need to include guidance on self-care in the treatment plan for individuals with CKD at any stage of the disease. It is also important to emphasise that family members are also affected by the disease, as they take on a significant burden of care. A structured family context plays an important role in the patient's process with morbidity, treatment and lifestyle changes (BARRETO, 2011).

In Portugal, integrated management applied to stage 5 chronic kidney disease has brought innovations in the way care is provided and patients on dialysis are monitored, with excellent results, demonstrating that CKD patients are satisfied and consider themselves to be properly informed and involved in decision-making about the choice of dialysis modality (COELHO, 2014).

Nozaki (2005) concludes in his study that self-care approaches are effective in increasing people's knowledge of CKD, controlling and recognising symptoms, and managing health status.

Previous studies have shown that some individuals recognise the importance of monitoring by nurses, as they are the professionals with whom they live most and develop a special relationship. This makes it possible for professionals to detect factors that may hinder adherence to treatment and to offer individualised support (LEWIS, 2010).

The role of the nursing team in the management of people with CKD, with the aim of avoiding complications, is reported by Travagim and Kusumota (2009). The authors highlight important guidelines such as combating smoking, alcohol, obesity and a sedentary lifestyle, as well as the need for access to medication, tests, establishing clinical guidelines and professional training. Rosol (2013) emphasises the need for screening and follow-up of people with cases of kidney disease in the family for early detection of new cases and better management.

Lewis (2010) emphasises the types of information people need at each stage of the disease. In the early stages, it is necessary to work on guidance about the disease, medications and self-care to preserve kidney function. In the more advanced stages, individuals need information about dietary changes, financial responsibilities and the types of treatment to replace kidney function.

Brogdon (2013) emphasises the importance of nurses in the process of health education and the need to make it accessible and relevant, providing care in a holistic way and respecting different levels of knowledge and beliefs, highlighting the responsibility of health control by CKD patients themselves, with professionals as advocates in helping them achieve well-being.

Clarkson's (2010) study found that lack of knowledge was the main factor in people's need for haemodialysis. The author highlights knowledge as the main tool for stabilising their state of health, but for this to happen, it is necessary to develop educational activities to reinforce changes in lifestyle that lead to improved results.

Santos, Rocha and Berardinelli (2011) carried out a study to assess the knowledge of CKD patients undergoing haemodialysis. The study shows that there are approximately 16 characteristics related to living with CKD: (time of discovery of the disease, recommended medical therapy, time spent on haemodialysis, physical exercise, leisure, diet); level of knowledge about living with renal replacement therapy (meaning of haemodialysis, forbidden foods, permitted foods, daily fluid consumption, care with venous access, complications with haemodialysis therapy, prevention of complications in haemodialysis, meaning of anticoagulation, post-hemodialysis symptoms, symptom control; meeting gregarious needs; interpersonal relationships). The authors concluded that the individuals needed guidance on self-care in almost all the aspects assessed, suggesting reinforced education and guidance work, especially on the part of the nursing team.

Silva (2013) proposes the implementation of waiting rooms in dialysis clinics as a space for health education in a critical and reflective way, working on co-responsibility and highlighting self-care as a means of change.

Carvalho and Santos (2009) suggest that the work of a multidisciplinary team contributes to adherence to treatment and is geared towards health promotion, as it provides conditions for achieving autonomy and encourages the exercise of citizenship.

It is important to emphasise that there are no tools for monitoring people with CKD. Tools are available for education, but not for recording and monitoring treatment.

Given the problem of the need for educational activities aimed at people with CKD, in order to achieve better control of the disease and its complications, this study aimed to build an educational technology for people with CKD and propose a tool for better recording information related to the treatment of CKD in order to accompany the individual to all appointments and make it easier for the health team to get to know the patient.

This study has produced a tool to help monitor the treatment of people with CKD, as well as containing important information about the disease, treatment, fluid intake, healthy lifestyle habits, dietary guidelines and legislation related to the disease. The technology allows any professional who cares for the individual to have information about their general state of health and the treatment they are undergoing, as well as containing information about CKD.

Technologies are concrete processes that, based on everyday experience and research, can develop a set of activities that will be produced and controlled by human beings. They can be conveyed as artefacts or as (structured) knowledge, systematised and with control over every step of the process. Technology then contributes to producing knowledge to be socialised, to mastering processes and products in order to transform empirical use into a scientific approach (educational technology in the school context) (GUBERT et al., 2009).

It is important to emphasise that not all technology is expensive. Normally, this is related to the expenditure of large sums of money. The technology proposed in this study is considered to be of low value and, as the professionals who analysed it have already pointed out, has good applicability.

CHAPTER 2

OBJECTIVES

2.1 General Objective

To describe the process of building and validating an educational technology for people with Chronic Kidney Disease.

2.2 Specific objectives

1) Validate the applicability of this educational technology with doctors and nurses who work with people with CKD;

2) Presenting a tool for recording information on CKD treatment.

CHAPTER 3

LITERATURE REVIEW

3.1 Chronic Kidney Disease

Chronic kidney disease (CKD) is a syndrome of progressive and irreversible loss of kidney function, the main causes of which are systemic arterial hypertension (SAH), diabetes mellitus (DM) and chronic glomerulonephritis (PERES, 2010).

According to the *National Kidney Disease Outcomes Quality Initiative* (NKF-K/DOQI), the diagnosis of CKD should be based on three components: anatomical or structural (markers of kidney damage), functional (based on the Glomerular Filtration Rate - GFR) and temporal. CKD is defined as the presence of markers of kidney damage for three months or more and the presence of GFR < 60 mL/min/1.73 m^2 or GFR > 60 mL/min/1.73 m2 associated with at least one marker of kidney damage (such as proteinuria and haematuria) for three months or more (K/DOQI, 2002).

Barbosa *et al.* (2006) point out that, in the terminal phase of the disease, the kidneys are no longer able to maintain the normality of the internal environment and, consequently, there is a loss of capacity for the excretion of toxic solutes by the kidneys, an inability to maintain the hydroelectrolytic and acid-base balance and systemic hormonal changes.

Sardenberg (2007) highlights the various causes of CKD, including primary renal diseases (chronic glomerulonephritis, chronic pyelonephritis, chronic tubulointerstitial nephritis and chronic obstructive diseases), systemic diseases (SAH, DM, autoimmune diseases, gout and amyloidosis), hereditary diseases (polycystic kidneys, Alport syndrome and cystinosis) and congenital malformations (renal agenesis, bilateral renal hypoplasia and posterior urethral valve).

The Ministry of Health also lists people at risk of developing CKD:

a) People with DM (either type 1 or type 2): the diagnosis of diabetes should be made based on a fasting serum glucose level above 126 mg/dL, or above 200 mg/dL 2 hours after ingesting 75g of glucose, or any value of hyperglycaemia, in the presence of classic symptoms such as polyuria, polydipsia or polyphagia;

b) People with SAH, defined as blood pressure values above 140/90 mmHg in two measurements 1 to 2 weeks apart;

c) Elderly people;

d)   Obese people (body mass index (BMI) > 30 Kg/m)$;^2$

e)   History of circulatory system disease (coronary heart disease, stroke, peripheral vascular disease, heart failure);

f)   Family history of CKD;

g)   Smoking;

h)   Use of nephrotoxic agents (BRASIL, 2014).

Generally, CKD progresses slowly and does not cause specific symptoms in the early stages. However, as it progresses, it mainly affects the gastrointestinal system (causing nausea and vomiting), the cardiovascular system (hypertension and oedema) and the haematological system (anaemia). These signs and symptoms are due to the retention of toxic solutes and/or excess action by homeostatic mechanisms (K/DOQI, 2002).

To assess kidney function, a widely used measure is the Glomerular Filtration Rate (GFR), estimated through 24-hour creatinine clearance. However, in some cases, due to collection errors or daily variations in creatinine excretion, this method may be lower than the estimates shown in the Glomerular Filtration Rate (GFR) equations. These differences occur mainly in amputees, vegetarians (who take creatinine supplements) and others (ROCHA, 2010).

The estimation of GFR in adults based on plasma creatinine can be calculated using the Crockcoft-Gault formula:

ClCr (ml/min) = (14 – idade) x peso (Kg) x (0,85 para mulheres)/ 72 x Cr plasmática (mg/dl)
Where: ClCr = creatinine clearance; plasma Cr = plasma creatinine

As the Crockcoft-Gault formula does not take body surface area into account, another formula used is that derived from the *Modification of Diet in Renal Disease* (MDRD) study:

FG (ml/min/1,73m²) = 1,86 x Creatser – 1154 x idade – 0.203 x (0,742 se mulher) (1,210 se negro)
Where: GF = Glomerular Filtration; Creatser = Serum Creatinine

The CKD-EPI (Chronic Kidney Disease Epidemiology Collaboration) sought to develop a more accurate equation, especially when GFR> 60 ml/min per 1.73 m^2 :

$$TFG = 141 \times \min(Scr/\kappa,1)^{a} \times \max(Scr/\kappa,1)^{-1.209} \times 0.993^{idade} \times 1.018 \text{ [se mulher]}$$

X 1.159

Where: Scr = serum creatinine; K= 0.7 for women and 0.9 for men; a = - 0.329 for women and - 0.411 for men

According to the assessment of kidney function, Riella (2010) presents the staging of CKD:

Chart 1 - Staging of Chronic Kidney Disease according to Riella (2010)

Internships	Description	FG (ml/min/1.73m2)
1	Kidney damage with normal or increased GF	≥ 90
2	Kidney damage with slightly decreased GF	60-89
3	Kidney damage with moderate decrease in GF	30-59
4	Kidney damage with severe decrease in GF	15-29
5	Renal failure, whether or not they are on dialysis	<15

People with a GFR between 30 and 45 ml/min, compared to those with a GFR > 60 ml/min, have a higher risk of mortality, up to 90 per cent, and cardiovascular mortality is around 110 per cent higher. For this reason, the most frightening clinical outcomes of CKD are cardiovascular disease, the need for renal replacement therapy (RRT) and all-cause mortality, especially cardiovascular mortality. Part of this context is the need to reinforce GFR control as a way of preventing CKD. This action has positive impacts and should be carried out (BRASIL, 2014).

Because it has no symptoms in the early stages, CKD requires health professionals, especially doctors, to sharpen its potential for suspicion, especially in people with risk factors. For this reason, Bastos and Kirsztjn (2011) suggest treatment based on three pillars of support:

1. Early diagnosis of the disease;

2. Immediate referral for nephrological treatment;

3. Implementation of measures to preserve kidney function.

Romão Júnior (2004) recommends dividing the treatment into a few components:

- **Health promotion and primary prevention programme (risk groups for CKD);**

- **Early identification of renal dysfunction (CKD diagnosis);**

- **Detection and correction of reversible causes of kidney disease;**

- **Aetiological diagnosis (type of kidney disease);**

- **Definition and staging of renal dysfunction;**

- **Institution of** interventions to slow down the progression of chronic kidney disease;

- **Prevent complications of chronic kidney disease;**

- **Modify** comorbidities common to these individuals;

- **Early planning of renal replacement therapy (RRT).**

The treatment of CKD depends on the progression of the disease and begins with conservative treatment (medication and diet, as well as control of underlying diseases) with the aim of keeping the person as long as possible without needing renal replacement therapy, as well as keeping them in good condition to start it when necessary (ROCHA, 2010). There are cases in which RRT (peritoneal dialysis, haemodialysis or transplantation) is necessary.

renal function), indicated when GFR is below 10 ml/min/1.73m, in addition to clinical and laboratory parameters.

The number of people with CKD undergoing RRT treatment has grown by around 7% a year worldwide. In Brazil, between 2000 and 2006, the number of people on dialysis grew by around 9% a year, and the Unified Health System (SUS) is responsible for 89% of the funding for this treatment (SZUSTER et al, 2012).

The Ministry of Health, in its Clinical Guidelines for the care of people with CKD, provides general recommendations for each stage of the disease (BRASIL, 2014):

Stages 1 and 2:

1. Reduce sodium intake (less than 2 g/day) corresponding to 5 g of sodium chloride in adults, unless contraindicated;
2. Physical activity compatible with cardiovascular health and tolerance: 30-minute walk 5 times a week to maintain BMI < 25;
3. Smoking cessation.

Stage 3[a] and 3B:

1. Reduce sodium intake (less than 2 g/day) corresponding to 5 g of sodium chloride in adults, unless contraindicated;
2. Physical activity compatible with cardiovascular health and tolerance: 30-minute walk 5 times a week to maintain BMI < 25;
3. Smoking cessation;

4. Correction of the dose of medications such as antibiotics and antivirals according to GFR.

<u>Stages 4 and 5:</u>

1. Reduce sodium intake (less than 2 g/day) corresponding to 5 g of sodium chloride, in adults, unless contraindicated;

4. Physical activity compatible with cardiovascular health and tolerance: 30-minute walk 5 times a week to maintain BMI < 25;

5. Smoking cessation;

6. Correction of the dose of medications such as antibiotics and antivirals according to GFR;

7. Reducing protein intake to 0.8 g/Kg/day in adults, accompanied by appropriate nutritional guidance, and avoiding intakes of more than 1.3 g/kg/day in individuals who require an intake of more than 0.8 g/kg/day for other reasons;

8. Oral bicarbonate replacement for people with metabolic acidosis, defined by a serum bicarbonate level below 22 mEq/L on venous blood gas analysis.

Travagim (2009) cites as public policies for the prevention of CKD the guidelines for the care offered to people on dialysis created in 2002 by the National Kidney Fundation (NKF), through the Disease Outcome Quality Initiative (DOQI), which emphasises the need for early diagnosis and follow-up in order to improve the health conditions of individuals entering RRT. Another policy mentioned by Travagim (2009) is the development of **the Ministry of Health's Primary Care** Notebook **"Clinical prevention of cardiovascular, cerebrovascular and renal diseases" with the aim of systematising the** recommended conduct based on scientific evidence.

It is important to publicise the "Clinical Guidelines for the Care of Patients with Chronic Kidney **Disease - CKD in the Unified Health System" established by the Ministry of Health in** 2014. These prescriptions aim to guide multi-professional teams in caring for people at risk of or diagnosed with CKD, covering risk stratification, prevention strategies, diagnosis and clinical management.

3.2 Haemodialysis

Dialysis is the term given to a type of treatment that aims to restore kidney function by removing toxic substances and excess water and mineral salts from the body, in an attempt to establish a balance. The term dialysis is used to refer to artificial or extrarenal blood purification, and is divided into: A) Haemodialysis (HD) and B) Peritoneal Dialysis (PD) (BRAGA, 2009).

Among the symptoms that indicate that dialysis treatment should be carried out in individuals in advanced stages are: symptoms of uremia (nausea, weakness, fatigue, disorientation, dyspnoea and oedema in the arms and legs), metabolic acidosis, hyperkalaemia and volume overload that are refractory to clinical treatment or when the GFR is below 10ml/min (TRAVAGIM AND KUSUMOTA, 2009; RIELLA 2010).

According to Szuster et *al.* (2012) the choice of RRT also depends on factors other than the individual and clinical characteristics of the person at the start of treatment, including: the preferences of individuals and doctors; geographical location and economic factors, such as how treatment is paid for and the availability of resources.

In Brazil, two types of dialysis are carried out: peritoneal dialysis and haemodialysis. Peritoneal dialysis is carried out in three different ways: intermittent dialysis (IPD), continuous ambulatory dialysis (CAPD) and automatic dialysis (APD); and standard haemodialysis (standard/status), which takes place three times a week for four hours a day, in different spaces, in hospitals/hospital satellite centres and in independent units/reference centres. It is important to note that home haemodialysis also exists in Brazil (dispensed six times a week for two hours a day), but it is not covered by the Unified Health System (SUS) (SANCHO and DAIN, 2008). In Brazil, haemodialysis is the most commonly performed RRT, accounting for 90% of dialyses (SZUSTER et *al.,* 2012).

According to Sesso et *al.* (2014), 73% of dialysis clinics in Brazil catered for people with chronic kidney disease undergoing conservative treatment and 67% for people with acute kidney injury. There has been an average annual increase in the number of individuals of 3% over the last 3 years. The prevalence rate of dialysis treatment in 2013 was 499 people per million population (pmp), varying by region from 284 pmp patients in the northern region to 622 pmp people in the southern region. The overall prevalence rate was stable compared to 2012 (503/pmp), which had shown growth of almost six per cent compared to 2011 (475/pmp). Fifty-five per cent of people (n = 18,700) started treatment in the Southeast, 6,019 individuals started dialysis in the Northeast, 5,249 in the South, 3,608 in the Centre-West and 1,668 in the North.

Riella (2010) reveals that haemodialysis became widespread as a treatment for chronic uremia in the 1960s, serving as an alternative to a disease that had been highly lethal until then. When it first appeared, it was used in cases of acute renal failure with the aim of keeping the individual alive until renal function recovered. Technological innovations have made it easier for the population to access this treatment, including improved machines, more efficient dialysers and surgical techniques for making permanent vascular accesses.

Haemodialysis is the process of filtering and purifying the blood, when the person's kidneys are unable to do so, of substances that need to be removed from the bloodstream, such as urea and creatinine (DAUGIRDAS *apud* ROCHA, 2010).

When two solutions are separated by a semi-permeable membrane, of the type used in haemodialysis, there is a bidirectional movement of the solute particles that are able to cross the membrane, there needs to be a difference in concentration between the solutions-diffusion, and there is also the same movement of the solvent, as there needs to be a difference in osmolarity-convection. The name dialysis is used for the process in which diffusion predominates, and urltrafiltration for the process in which convection predominates. Absorption (removal of solutes by the filters) is emphasised when the blood comes into contact with the membranes (RIELLA, 2010).

Rocha (2010) points out that haemodialysis requires venous access. This can be permanent (arteriovenous fistula - AVF) or temporary (double or triple lumen catheters). The AVF is performed in a surgical setting, almost always under local anaesthetic, preferably in the non-dominant limb with anastomosis between the radial artery and cephalic vein, brachial and cephalic or brachial and basilic. Catheters can be implanted in the subclavian, internal jugular and femoral veins. The jugular vein is the most popular, as it has the fewest complications.

During haemodialysis, blood must come into contact with the walls of the extracorporeal circuit, but no matter how advanced the machines, using biocompatible materials, they are still thrombogenic. Hence the need to use an anticoagulant (except in cases of clinical contraindications) to prevent obstruction of the circuit, as well as reducing the loss of internal volume of the dialyser fibres, maintaining the efficiency of the equipment. The most commonly used anticoagulant is unfractionated heparin due to its low cost, ease of use, short half-life and the possibility of neutralising it (ROCHA, 2010).

Nascimento and Marques (2015) point out that the complications that occur during haemodialysis sessions can be casual, but some can be extremely serious and even fatal. In descending order of frequency, the most common are: hypotension (20%-30% of dialyses), cramps (5%-20%), nausea and vomiting (5%-15%), headache (5%), chest pain (2%-5%), low back pain (2%-5%), pruritus (5%), fever and chills (< 1%). Less common but serious complications that can cause death include: imbalance syndrome, hypersensitivity reactions, arrhythmia, intracranial haemorrhage, convulsions, haemolysis and gas embolism.

In addition to occasional complications during dialysis treatment, the comorbidity of individuals is high and is associated with cardiovascular diseases, systemic arterial hypertension, anaemia, susceptibility to infection, type B and C hepatitis, bone diseases, malnutrition and other less well-defined causes (BARBOSA et al., 2006).

CKD sufferers need to be advised about: the disease itself; treatment; forms of renal replacement therapy and the risks and benefits associated with each; vascular access; early dialysis access (arteriovenous fistula or peritoneal dialysis catheter); diet; water restriction; medication use; blood pressure and glycaemia control (SANTOS; ROCHA; BERARDINELLI, 2011). It is recommended that CKD patients in stage 4 receive guidance on RRT and the necessary care. The Ministry of Health makes the following recommendations for individuals on dialysis (BRASIL, 2014):

Internship 5D- in dialysis:

1. Reduce sodium intake (less than 2 g/day) corresponding to 5 g of sodium chloride in adults, unless contraindicated;

2. Physical activity compatible with cardiovascular health and tolerance: 30-minute walk 5 times a week to maintain BMI < 25;

3.   Smoking cessation;

4. Correction of the dose of medications such as antibiotics and antivirals according to the dialysis modality;

5. Adequacy of protein intake according to nutritional status, assessment of hyperphosphataemia and adequacy of dialysis.

For people undergoing dialysis treatment, the lack of knowledge about changes resulting from the therapy is an important stress factor (BARRETO, 2011). Studies show that individuals themselves have concerns about their health situation, such as grafts and fistulas, catheter insertion, treatment options and the use of prescribed medication (LEWIS, 2010). There are frequent doubts that are part of the renal patient's daily life and require the participation of the professional and the family in the treatment and comprehensive monitoring. The most **recurrent** doubts **are about: "food allowed"; test results; procedures; the** need or not for a transplant (QUEIROZ, 2008).

Kidney patients can feel hopeless as they carry the weight of a chronic illness, especially when they need dialysis. In this way, they become vulnerable to the complications that the disease brings, as they need special attention that requires obligations and renunciations, as well as frequent demands for self-care. In addition, there are difficulties related to job instability, often due to absenteeism; decreased self-esteem and sexual activity, due to neurological, endocrine, psychological, biochemical, pharmacological and haematological factors. All of these factors reinforce the premise of the need for comprehensive and close care for CKD patients (FORTES,

2013).

The feeling of dependence on a machine can awaken a sense of grief in kidney patients. This is yet another factor that points to the importance of raising awareness about the disease and treatment, so that they feel motivated and encouraged to change certain behaviours that can be harmful to their health.

Breitsameter (2008) lists complications related to people with CKD seeking emergency care, including dyspnoea, respiratory system infections, fever, neurological changes, sensory changes and convulsions, changes in blood pressure levels, bleeding (digestive and nasal), nausea and vomiting, low back pain, complications from arteriovenous fistulas (AVFs), precordialgia and anaemia.

As the main concern is the CKD patient's quality of life and the nurse is the professional in closest and most constant contact with this individual, Mariane and Fortes *(apud* ROCHA, 2010) highlight the nurse's role in preparing for RRT and when the person starts therapy:

Preparation for RRT:

• Introduce the person/family member to all the dialysis options and methods so that they can choose the one that best suits their lifestyle (taking into account the clinical indications);

•		Provide access (AVF or catheter);

• Encouraging the individual to attend appointments with a psychologist for assessment and treatment of emotional aspects that may interfere with their quality of life;

• Arrange an initial interview with a social worker to identify socio-economic conditions and the social security situation;

• Strictly monitor GFR to ensure that the person is in good condition for the start of RRT;

• Educate the individual to recognise signs of malnutrition, volume overload and other uremic symptoms;

• Advise the person to go to a healthcare professional when they notice a change in their state of health and to avoid urgent dialysis.

When the person starts RRT:

• Determine the start date and the days of the week and times of haemodialysis according to the individual's lifestyle;

• Accompanying the person to the haemodialysis sessions and communicating with the nephrologist to adjust the individualised medical prescription;

• Observe the AVF limb at every session in order to detect stenoses, aneurysms, pseudo-aneurysms or infections at an early stage;

• Train and supervise the nursing team to rotate AVF puncture sites (in order to avoid weakening the vessel and consequently aneurysms);

• Record nursing actions and interventions in medical records.

Given all the difficulties faced by CKD patients undergoing haemodialysis, Carvalho (2009) stresses the need for health professionals to be prepared to answer questions and to always be aware of the importance of professional-user interaction.

In addition, Morante et al (2014) highlight the need for professionals to be aware of the interval between the individual's diagnosis and the length of time they have been on dialysis, in order to provide more appropriate care and guidance, as these variables affect the way in which each case should be handled.

The role of the nurse is of paramount importance in this process of orientating the individual, because although educating the client with CKD is a commitment of the entire health team, this professional works more constantly and more closely with this clientele (SANTOS; ROCHA; BERARDINELLI, 2011).

3.3 Health Education for Chronic Kidney Disease Patients

Health education is a dynamic process aimed at empowering people to improve their health conditions. It is important to note that the people taking part can accept or reject the guidelines for changing their behaviour. In order for it to develop and be successful, it is not enough to impose rules on individuals on how to be healthier and avoid illnesses, but rather to carry out education based on dialogue, enquiry and reflection, so that this educational intervention can contribute to changes in lifestyle and encourage the prevention and/or control of illnesses, resulting in a better quality of life (MARTINS; CESARINO, 2007).

Carvalho and Gastaldo (2008) point out that, through empowerment, health promotion seeks to provide individuals and groups with learning that makes them capable of living life at all stages and living with the limitations imposed by some illnesses, suggesting that these actions should be carried out in different environments, including school, home, work and community groups.

Health education is a set of knowledge and practices that aim to prevent illness and promote health. For health education activities to be successful, it is necessary to get to know users, their habits, beliefs and the conditions in which they live (ALVEZ, 2005).

One advantage of this educational activity is that it is low cost and easy to carry out, as well as being able to be carried out from primary to tertiary care. The participation of the agents in a joint and constructive way, i.e. professionals and people with chronic diseases, as well as the family, is essential for effective actions to be taken to improve health care.

Favé (2014) emphasises that health education helps people acquire knowledge and skills to deal with the disease. The study carried out in France assessed a group of 80 patients with stage 3 CKD (non-dialysis treatment) and asked them if they were interested in taking part in a health education programme called the Therapeutic Education Programme. Of these, 30 refused to take part, citing reasons such as lack of interest, difficulty in getting to the clinic due to the distance, being very old and having other interests. The author of the article highlights the importance of the multidisciplinary team in the acceptance of health education and when they have it, they accept participation in education programmes better.

Martins and Cesarino (2004) highlight a number of programmes for the education and rehabilitation of individuals with kidney disease, among them:

- Life Options Rehabilitation Advisory Council, is a multidisciplinary programme created in 1994 by the Institute of Medical Education, United States, which offers technical support and develops educational materials, based on encouragement, education, exercise, employment and evaluation, for all kidney patients and professionals in the field.

It is a national programme that is particularly active in three areas: rehabilitation, programmes and publications, and research into renal rehabilitation.

- Educational Programme 1 - was a pilot follow-up study carried out in Sweden, which recruited people with chronic kidney disease regardless of treatment modality, gender and age. They took a course in their homes and were assessed before and after the course by comparing data. All participants persisted in emotional stability and increasing functional capacity.

- Life Readiness Program - a physical rehabilitation programme for people on haemodialysis, conducted by the Department of Nephrology and Hypertension in Chapel

Hill, North Carolina, United States. It observed an improvement in sleep, a reduction in dialysis-related symptoms and changes in the lifestyle of CKD patients and carers.

Studies have shown an improvement in the behaviour, self-management and quality of life of people who are accompanied by professionals who carry out health education, but they report a temporary improvement, i.e. only while they are being accompanied. Once they had to carry out self-care and self-manage their lifestyle, these gains diminished (NOZAKI, 2005). These results are reinforced by Karavetian (2014) who reports working with individuals who received guidance on diet and were monitored, showing significant improvements in the progression of the disease and in quality of life.

Silva (2012) lists the main conditions that can interfere with adherence to CKD treatment, among them: acceptance of the disease; level of education; stable emotional relationships (family and friends); side effects; long period and complex treatment regimen; lack of access to medication; trust in the team and absence of symptoms, as well as psychological, demographic, nutritional and socioeconomic factors.

Greer, Crews and Boulware (2012) also highlight barriers that can hinder health education for people with CKD, including an inadequate multidisciplinary approach in primary care, a lack of infrastructure and support for education activities.

Araújo et al. (2014) report on the work carried out through campaigns with the aim of screening individuals with risk factors for CKD, informing them about the disease and referring them for follow-up and analysing the data collected, with the aim of generating a panel on CKD in Ceará. This action contributes to the formulation of recommendations for prevention that include improved surveillance, screening, education, warning and awareness of people at risk of developing the disease.

World Kidney Day has been taking place since 2006 as a joint initiative of the International Society of Nephrology (ISN) and the International Federation of Kidney Foundations (IFKF) and aims to raise awareness of the importance of the kidneys for general health and to reduce the frequency and impact of kidney disease and associated health problems worldwide. Each year, the campaign addresses a topic for discussion, providing information and sample materials on its own website (http://www.worldkidneyday.com).

Choi and Lee (2012) carried out a study using the "face-to-face" methodology, which consisted of individual or small group meetings with the intention of orientating and educating people with CKD about their disease and treatment. They obtained an improvement in the participating group's knowledge of the disease itself and treatment one week after the meetings began.

Nunes (2013) emphasises that when education begins from the first encounter, there is a greater likelihood of involvement and understanding of the disease. So she developed and applied an instrument for the first consultation with the nephrologist, working on the pathophysiology of the disease as a form of guidance and education to prevent and delay the progression of the disease.

Cesarino and Casagrande (1998) carried out an action research project observing individuals on haemodialysis based on their behaviour during treatment and listed themes to be worked on in subsequent educational activities. They concluded that, with educational activities developed using the awareness-raising methodology, it was possible to provide reflection and understanding of the basic elements regarding the reality of the disease and the therapeutic regimens used. These findings corroborate the results of the study by Murphy et *al.* (2008), who concluded that educating CKD patients and their families is fundamental, as it allows them to make informed choices and prevents complications.

Silva (2013) highlights the waiting room as a potential territory for exchanging experiences, as it allows people to experience more intensely or not the same dilemmas, doubts, difficulties and happiness. These interactions can be considered a moment of convergence between popular and technical-scientific knowledge.

Freitas et al. (2011) point out that health education in the Basic Health Unit should not be limited to one-off, scheduled situations, but should always take place naturally during consultations, as the Unit is a fertile ground for education activities because it is in constant contact with the individual and their family.

A randomised intervention study showed that a specific nutritional education programme with chronic kidney disease patients in stages 3 to 5 was able to reduce protein intake when compared to standard dietary advice (PAES-BARRETO et al., 2013). The US Department of Agriculture has developed a tool called MyPlate to work on nutritional education with chronic kidney disease patients through the image of a plate containing the food group and the amounts that people should eat (PROSCIA, 2014). Mancini et al. (2012), in a study carried out in Italy with 97 CKD patients undergoing conservative treatment, investigated the effectiveness of education in the pre-dialysis period. After the educational measures, most of the individuals (79%) had a good level of knowledge about haemodialysis and peritoneal dialysis. The authors concluded that the guidance given to people before starting dialysis treatment helps them choose the type of treatment and facilitates adherence. This same study found that 53 per cent of people did not have sufficient knowledge about kidney function and the need for other therapies (erythropoietin, vitamin D and antihypertensive drugs).

An intensified nutritional education programme, carried out in São José dos Campos-SP, resulted in an improvement in individuals' knowledge of various aspects related to the control of hyperkalaemia and was associated with a significant reduction in serum potassium concentrations (VASCONCELLOS; BRAGA; SOAR, 2012).

Education and health promotion activities developed in groups can be a possibility for raising the level of knowledge, acceptance of their limits and awareness of positive attitudes (SILVA, 2013). It also favours the individual's participation in deciding their own fate and acting to improve their quality of life.

It is important that educational programmes help with treatment, making people understand the disease and contributing to their emotional and functional well-being. Stimulating adherence to treatment and reducing morbidity and mortality during treatment are objectives of the educational approach (GRICIO, KUSUMOTA and CÂNDIDO, 2009).

Sally (2012) highlights the importance of constant training for professionals to prevent complications related to haemodialysis, including infections. Strategies to prevent complications through diet, guidance on renal replacement therapies and symptom management are emphasised as important roles for professionals working with these individuals (LEWIS, 2010).Greer, Crews and Boulware (2012) cite testimonies from primary care professionals who say they are unprepared to educate people with CKD because they don't have enough knowledge about the disease and, when they do, they report other obstacles such as their low level of education.

3.4 Educational Technologies

Rocha (2008) refers to technology as a set of abstract and concrete actions with purposes, which permeates the entire health work process. Educational technologies are used to make health work processes a reality. Health technologies include: medicines, equipment and technical procedures, organisational, educational, information and support systems and care programmes and protocols, through which health care is provided to the population (MAGALHÃES; SANTOS, 2009).

Technologies can be classified and divided into soft (dealing with relationships), yeast (referring to well-structured knowledge, for example, the nursing process) and hard (covering technological equipment such as machines, as well as standards (MERHY, 2002).

Research must go beyond the conceptual and methodological and contribute to the solution of existing problems, thus improving the quality of care and implementing more effective policies. But in order to use technology as an aid to the care process, professionals need to be attentive to individualised, dynamic care with a range of possibilities for gaining the patient's trust and commitment to improving their quality of life.

Scientific policies have expanded the search for knowledge and innovations in many countries, seeking to understand the problem and, most importantly, to contribute to quality health care for the population, consequently generating economic growth for the country when this scientific production is articulated with other strategic social sectors (GUIMARÃES, 2013).

Carneiro (2014) recounts the progress of discussions and productions related to health technologies since the 1990s, when the Ministry of Health sought to strengthen the Unified Health System (SUS) through the Strengthening the Reorganisation of the SUS (REFORSUS) project, financed by the World Bank and the Inter-American Development Bank (IDB) with the intention of acquiring medical and hospital equipment, as well as improving management, which included technological assessment. Between 2003 and 2004, a working group was set up within the Science, Technology and Innovation Council of the Ministry of Health. In 2005, the Secretariat for Science and Technology and Strategic Inputs (SCTIE) was created, responsible for implementing and disseminating health technology actions in the SUS. In 2008, the Brazilian Network for Health Technology Assessment (REBRATS) was set up to bring academic institutions and health services closer together. In recent years, Brazil has still faced difficulties and obstacles, but has made significant progress in the science, technology and innovation (S&T&I) sector.

Brogdon (2013) cites the difficulties that professionals have in guiding people on haemodialysis to an appropriate diet as a source of frustration, as he has noticed a low rate of adherence. In addition to diet, water intake must also be adjusted to avoid possible complications (NOZAKI, 2005). These and many other authors cite the countless difficulties of working with individuals who have a low level of education or when the disease itself ends up limiting the patient's knowledge due to the complexity and difficulty of coping with it.

It is therefore believed that educational work with groups is an important alternative for Educational Technology in Health, aimed at promoting health and deepening discussions and knowledge, enabling people to improve their level of autonomy and, consequently, their quality of life (CARNEIRO, 2014).

Diamantidis (2013) demonstrates the use of a strategy to educate people with chronic kidney disease on risks related to their health condition through a website where they can learn a little more about the disease, clarify doubts and recognise risk actions for complications.

In order to work with educational technologies in health, it is necessary to have trained professionals who not only have knowledge about the disease, but also have the skills to develop the technologies and use effective pedagogical strategies to work with individuals. Carneiro (2014) emphasises the importance of the role of nurses in this process, as they work at different levels of health care (including different levels of prevention).

Rodrigues (2011) says that there is a lot of information about CKD in books and on the internet, but when he spoke to people with the disease, he realised that they wanted to know more about their condition. That's why he produced a booklet for kidney patients with guidance on various topics related to CKD, such as the pathophysiology of the disease, diet, legislation, treatment and more. The booklet, which is available online, also provides guidance on the possibility of needing to retire if the individual is unable to work.

Jacopetti (2011) describes field research with the public linked to a philanthropic organisation for the treatment of kidney patients that had recently undergone the process of technological convergence towards web 2.0. It was concluded that the virtual environment is a space for interaction and dissemination of information on the prevention of kidney diseases, health and quality of life issues, sending news and interviews, sharing stories of kidney patients, among other subjects, demonstrating the relevance of yet another educational technology in health.

Gaubert et al. (2009) report on their experience working with adolescents in a municipal school in Fortaleza-CE. In the project, the adolescents themselves developed a light technology to work on sexual and reproductive health.

Santos and Lima (2005) used health education technology to assess lifestyle changes among university workers through monthly workshops, seeking to assess participants' knowledge of hypertension and then work on ways of educating them to adopt healthy lifestyle habits.

Various websites provide guidance for kidney patients on diet, medication, healthy habits, events related to the subject and news. Among them are: Portal da diálise- educar para prevenir (http://www.portaldadialise.com); Pró-Renal- com você fazemos mais pela vida (http://www.pro-renal.org.br); Pró-Rim (http://www.prorim.org.br); Amigos do Rim (http://www.amigosdorim.com.br); Fundação do Rim- semeando superação (http://www.flindacaodorimce.org.br).

In view of the above, the importance of working in health through educational technologies is emphasised, as it allows for the participation of the patient and the professionals involved, as well as promoting health through the search for healthy lifestyle habits based on knowledge of the disease, the risks and practices to improve quality of life.

CHAPTER 4

METHODOLOGY

4.1 Type of research

This is a descriptive methodological study to build an educational technology and a tool for recording information related to the treatment of CKD. Polit, Beck and Hungler (2004) conceptualise a methodological study as one that investigates, organises and analyses data in order to construct, validate and evaluate research instruments and techniques, focusing on the development of specific data collection tools with a view to improving the reliability and validity of these instruments. A mixed-methods study was also carried out, using both qualitative and quantitative methods.

4.2 Study phases

The study was carried out in dialysis clinics located in the city of Fortaleza-Ceará, where there are currently 13 dialysis centres. These centres provide specialised care for people with CKD undergoing dialysis and conservative (non-dialysis) treatment. The participating clinics were: Instituto de Nefrologia do Ceará (INECE), Prontorim S/C Ltda, Instituto do Rim Ltda, Pronefron Ltda- Filial Messejana, Instituo de Doenças Renais Ltda and Policlínica do Rim S/C Ltda. These centres treat an average of 170 individuals per month.

Professionals (doctors and nurses) who had been working with CKD patients in dialysis centres for at least two years and who agreed to take part in the research were interviewed. A total of 12 professionals took part.

A large number of professionals refused to take part in the research, claiming that they lacked the time to evaluate the Educational Technology Proposal (ETP).

Data was collected in October 2015 by presenting the TPP (Appendix 3) and the TPP evaluation questionnaire (Appendix 4) initially to the directors of the clinics (with the signing of the Letter of Consent) through a conversation highlighting the importance of the research and the collaboration of those involved.

Subsequently, contact was made with the professionals (doctors and nurses).

Initially, they were informed about the objectives and methodology used for the study and then the technology was presented, with any doubts clarified. The TPP presented to the professionals can be seen in Chart 2 (Appendix 3).

The documents were then distributed: Invitation letter (Appendix 1); Informed Consent Form (ICF) (Appendix 2) in two copies; PTE (Appendix 3) and PTE evaluation questionnaire (with objective and subjective questions) (Appendix 4).

4.3 Data processing and analysis

The data contained in the instruments answered by the participants was organised and processed in an Excel spreadsheet, represented in tables and charts. The results were analysed using analytical and descriptive statistics.

After gathering the evaluations carried out by the doctors and nurses, it was realised that the format in which the PTE was presented and the information it contained would not bring the desired results in terms of monitoring and evaluating people with CKD. This led to the idea of producing a tool that would make this monitoring possible, as is already done with pregnant women and children, for example.

Research was carried out to find out what already exists in terms of monitoring tools for people with CKD, examples of monitoring tools and the information that would need to be included in the booklet.

Caderneta was then produced using the Corel Draw X7 programme, combining vector elements (drawings) and text. Initially, the concept of format (size) and colour that best suited the booklet's user audience was considered. From there, the texts were laid out and the images produced.

4.6 Ethical and legal aspects

The research was carried out in accordance with Resolution 466/2012 of the National Research Ethics Commission (CONEP/CNS/MS) (Brazil, 2012), which regulates research with human beings. Participants were informed about the nature and objectives of the research and anonymity, and it was emphasised that they could withdraw their consent whenever they wished. Data collection was carried out after signing the Informed Consent Form (ICF) and receiving a favourable opinion from the Ethics and Research Committee (CEP) of the University of Fortaleza - UNIFOR under number 1.325.983.

CHAPTER 5

RESULTS

The results presented are based on the Educational Technology Proposal (ETP) that was evaluated by the doctors and nurses who took part in the research.

Chart 2 - Educational Technology Proposal (ETP) - Prevention of complications arising from Chronic Kidney Disease.

PREVENTIVE AND/OR CONTROL MEASURES FOR COMPLICATIONS RESULTING FROM CHRONIC KIDNEY DISEASE
Nutrition
Adequate salt and sugar intake Avoid sausages and tinned food; Avoid foods high in sugar; Remove the salt shaker from the table; Reduce the amount of salt in food preparation; Use natural spices (garlic, onion, chives, bay leaves, basil, oregano, pepper, parsley, vinegar, etc.).
Fluid intake Control your intake of water, coffee, soft drinks, tea, milk, broths and soups.
Protein intake Choose meat, chicken, fish or eggs for lunch and dinner.
Vegetable fat intake Favour vegetable cream, margarine or unsalted butter.
Potassium intake Cook vegetables (cauliflower, spinach, aubergine, green beans, okra, broccoli, courgettes, potatoes, cassava and pumpkin) in water and discard the cooking water.
Preference for vegetables Give preference to fruit and vegetables; Do not eat star fruit or drink its natural juice.
Blood pressure and glycaemic control
Blood pressure Measure blood pressure weekly.
Blood sugar Carry out periodic examinations in accordance with medical advice.
Habits
Smoking Avoid using cigarettes and other drugs (cannabis, crack, cocaine).
Alcoholism

Avoid drinking alcoholic beverages.
Regular physical exercise   Carry out exercise according to medical advice and guidance.
Adequate sleep and rest   Sleep (8 to 10 hours a night);   Rest (2 to 3 hours a day).
Stress management   Search for leisure options   Look for social support that helps reduce stress (groups, associations).   Follow spiritual guidelines that you believe in and that bring relief from anxieties and fears.
Systematic attendance at appointments   Always be present at scheduled appointments (medical or nursing) and haemodialysis sessions.
Medication
The risk of self-medication   Only use prescribed medication.
Regular use of prescribed medication (if applicable)   Take the medicine exactly as prescribed.
Dialysis
Knowledge of the procedure   Clarify doubts about dialysis whenever they arise.
Transplant
Seek information on the indications for transplantation and precautions to avoid the need for this procedure.

Characterisation of Employees

Twelve professionals working in dialysis centres were interviewed, 7 nurses (58.3%) and 5 doctors (41.7%). The participants had a mean age of 35±8.3 years (ranging from 26 to 53 years) and 58.3% were female. The average length of training was 9.5±7.7 years (ranging from 2 to 28 years), while the length of time working in nephrology was 7.9±5.7 years (ranging from 2 to 20 years). All of the interviewees had a postgraduate qualification in Nephrology (with one in progress). The distribution of interviewees according to socio-demographic and professional data is summarised in Table 1.

Table 1- Distribution of interviewees according to sociodemographic and professional data. Fortaleza, CE, 2015.

Personal and Professional Data n=12	n	%	Average Standard

	n	%	Mean	deviation
Professional category: Nurses	7	58,3	-	-
Doctors	5	41,7	-	-
Age	-	-	35	8,3
Gender: Female	7	58,3	-	-
Male	5	41,7	-	-
Training time	-	-	9,5	7,7
Time in Professional Practice	-	-	9,5	7,5
Time working in Nephrology	-	-	7,9	5,7
Postgraduate studies in Nephrology	12	100	-	-

Evaluation of the Educational Technology Proposal (ETP)

The professionals' assessment of the TPP was divided into the following aspects:

1. Feasibility/Applicability

When assessing the feasibility and applicability of the ETP, 9 (75 per cent) of the professionals said it was a technology that could be used.

> *"Extremely important, especially in an area of health where the population has little knowledge, as do professionals from other areas"*
>
> *"It seems to me to be a simple way that's easy to apply and has potentially good results"*
>
> *"Very useful, providing better guidance for patients"*
>
> *"I think it's feasible and applicable because it's an easy and objective tool that doesn't bore the professional or the patient or take up too much time."*
>
> *"I think it's extremely important and timely due to the range of complications witnessed in haemodialysis rooms and the lack of information"*

Some professionals (25 per cent) didn't think it was feasible to apply the TEP.

> *"The way it's described, I don't think it's viable, reading documents doesn't attract their attention. I believe that the nutritional content should be covered by a nutritionist. Review the approach to transplantation"*
>
> *"Little applicability, as leaflets are generally not read by patients. "*
>
> *"I believe that patients are resistant to changing their behaviour (habits) and diet. "*

2. Approach to preventive behaviour

According to 8 of the participants (66.6%), the TPP addresses preventive behaviours for CKD.

> *"It's a very rich table, which covers various aspects. "*
>
> *"It contains very important guidelines, but lacks guidance on access care (catheter and arteriovenous fistula)."*

3. Does it help professionals to prevent complications from CKD?

According to the majority of participants (75 per cent), the TPP makes an important contribution to the work of professionals in preventing complications arising from CKD.

"Helps the professional pin down the main aspects to be discussed with the patient. " "Helps with treatment follow-up and makes the professional remember the patient's restrictions."

4. Does it help people to seek measures to prevent CKD complications?

Most of the participants (83.3%) reported that the TPP was very important for the individual in terms of changing habits, adapting to treatment and improving quality

of life. It was also suggested that the project be extended to outpatient clinics and not restricted to dialysis centres.

"Of paramount importance for the patient in raising awareness of nutritional status and preventing comorbidities. "

"I believe that the more the patient is orientated in relation to the treatment, the more likely they are to follow the guidelines and carry out the treatment correctly. "

"It's an important tool for the patient to know and accept the restrictions and clear up any doubts. "

"The use of this technology would lead to a significant reduction in hospitalisations and mortality. "

"It contributes to improving the quality of life of these patients. "

Table 2 - Evaluation of the TPP by professionals. Fortaleza, CE, 2015. n=12

Aspects	YES		NO	
	n	**%**	**n**	**%**
Is it feasible/applicable?	9	75	3	25
Does it include preventive behaviour?	8	66,6	4	33,3
Helps professionals prevent/control complications ?	9	75	3	25
Does it help the individual to prevent/control complications?	10	83,3	2	16,6

5. Suggestions for changes to the TPP:

5.1 Scope

With regard to the scope of the TPP, some suggestions were made, including: emphasising young people; adding guidance for carers and involving the multidisciplinary team (especially the nutritionist).

"In this format, it's limited to those who read."

"It's important to apply a questionnaire to carers as well."

5.2 Contents

It was suggested that the following aspects be added to the content of the ETP: the importance of time and attendance at haemodialysis sessions; risks so that primary and secondary prevention is more effective; venous access for haemodialysis; skin, ophthalmological, endocrine, muscular and gynaecological lesions and nephrotoxic drugs; vaccination; serology.

"It's important to include risk factors so that primary and secondary prevention can be started early."

Include the main nephrotoxic drugs.

"Addressing lesions in various areas such as: skin, ophthalmological, endocrine, muscular and gynaecological.

"To provide patients and staff with knowledge about monitoring dialysis treatment. "

"Include an approach to social issues, benefits, retirement. "

5.3 Objectivity

There were no suggestions for changes to the PTE's objectivity.

5.4 Structure

Regarding the structure of the PTE, the professionals suggested that it should give professionals the chance to get to know complicated situations, as well as using images.

"The way it is presented, as a leaflet, it may not be the right structure for the patient to absorb the information, as they may not be interested. " "Leaflets are not usually read by patients. " "It's important to include images. "

5.5 Language

With regard to the language presented in the TEP, the majority of participants said they would not change it, as they believe that the language presented is already clear, objective and accessible to people with CKD. Only one participant said that the language was not appropriate, but did not suggest any changes.

"The language is clear and objective. "

"Accessible to patients."

"Simple and practical, allowing the content to be understood. "

Table 3 - Aspects to be modified according to the opinion of the professionals.

Fortaleza - CE. n=12

Aspects	YES		NO	
	n	%	n	%
Scope	7	58,3	5	41,6
Contents	5	41,6	7	58,3
Objectivity	2	16,6	10	83,3
Structure	3	25	9	75
Language	2	16,6	10	83,3

6. Other suggestions

The participants also highlighted other suggestions for changes to improve the TPP.

"Extend the project to outpatient clinics providing conservative treatment for CKD and not restrict it to haemodialysis centres

in order to mitigate the problem of late referrals to dialysis centres. "

"Involve the multi-professional team. "

"Nutritional guidance can be individualised with the participation of a nutritionist. " "Mention and emphasise the carer, who we often forget, whether a family member or not, is of fundamental importance to the patient's treatment and the prevention of comorbidities. "

It should be emphasised that all the suggestions made by the participating professionals were of great value to the production of the educational technology and contributed to the creation of the Renal Patient Handbook.

It was from analysing the professionals' evaluations of the TPP that the intention arose to produce a technology that would include important guidelines for CKD patients, but which would also be a tool for professionals to monitor these individuals and take on a role of identity for chronic kidney disease patients.

CHAPTER 6

DISCUSSION

The need for early diagnosis and prevention of complications was reinforced by almost all the participants in this survey, who believe that TEP helps people to seek measures to prevent comorbidities, to be made aware of the importance of eating habits that jeopardise their state of health, to accept restrictions, to seek healthy lifestyle habits and, consequently, to increase the quality of life of CKD sufferers.

Riella (2010) presents all the care that should be carried out with kidney patients from the beginning of the discovery of the disease in order to prevent its progression and to prevent complications such as anaemia, bone-mineral disease, dyslipidaemia, hypertension, malnutrition, among others. The author presents the clinical management of CKD patients at all stages of the disease and highlights the need for RRT depending on the GFR value, the presence and intensity of signs and symptoms of uremia, as well as the availability of RRT and the individual's preference.

Bastos (2011) highlights one of the pillars of CKD treatment as the immediate referral of people for follow-up by a nephrologist or nephrology team, which also reduces costs when treatment is started early. When discovered early on, the disease can be treated conservatively and, depending on the indications, RRT may be necessary, which includes haemodialysis, peritoneal dialysis and kidney transplantation.

The evaluation of the PTE indicated that most of the participants believe that it contributes to the professional's work in preventing complications arising from CKD to the extent that it reminds them of the main aspects to be addressed during consultations, as well as helping the professional to highlight each person's restrictions.

In order to prevent the individual from needing RRT, in addition to early diagnosis, special care is needed for self-care, including guidance on medication adherence, avoiding nephrotoxic drugs and diet control. The suggestions made by the survey participants emphasised the importance of these guidelines, as well as care with vascular access, fluid intake and relevant legislation.

Nunes et *al.* (2011) concluded in a study that knowledge about the disease improved self-management in haemodialysis patients, improved glycaemic control in people with diabetes and adherence to treatment in people with HIV.

Murphy et al. (2008) emphasise the difficulty chronic kidney patients have in following guidelines, such as major liquid and dietary restrictions. For this reason, the authors stress the importance of educating patients and carers as a way of minimising these difficulties through guidance on the disease, treatment and care needed. This corroborates the suggestions made by the participants in this survey, in which most professionals highlighted the lack of information the population has about kidney disease and the importance of educating CKD patients, including those undergoing haemodialysis, as it is a procedure that is so prone to complications due to a lack of information.

An instrument was produced to assess kidney patients' knowledge about CKD and showed that there is a lack of knowledge about many aspects related to self-care that are not well understood by individuals (NUNES et al., 2011). This conclusion reinforces the opinion of many professionals who have evaluated the TPP and stated that there is a huge lack of information, not only from patients, but also from carers and professionals from other areas, and that the more information that is passed on, the more likely the person is to follow the guidelines of the team that accompanies them.

Several studies have shown the importance of health education in improving CKD patients' adherence to treatment. Porter (2013) presented good results in an educational study with pre-dialysis CKD patients, which helped to extend dialysis time and reduce hospitalisations. The study showed that people with pre-dialysis educational interventions survived 8 months longer and indicated that conventional approaches are inadequate, because in order to be an active participant, the individual needs to be sufficiently informed and have the autonomy and responsibility to make decisions about treatment.

Another study, carried out by Tamura et al. (2014), highlighted the improvement in some clinical domains presented by individuals who underwent counselling, among them the greater survival of patients after starting dialysis. Caldeira et al. (2011) reported improved control of serum phosphorus levels in people on dialysis who underwent education and/or counselling. Rioux et al. (2011) point out that educational intervention influences the patient's choice of treatment modality, as they become more knowledgeable about the subject and feel responsible for the treatment they are going to undergo.

Choi and Lee (2012) carried out an educational intervention with individuals before RRT, with individual guidance involving doctors, nurses and nutritionists, and found that the intervention improved people's knowledge of CKD and their self-care.

All these studies reinforce the importance of health education for people with CKD, stressing that they need guidance right from the start, because the sooner people are made aware of health care, including restrictions, the less likely they are to have complications from the disease, reducing the number of hospitalisations and even death, according to the opinion of the professionals who trialled the technology proposed in this study. The study carried out by Huang and Carrero (2014) highlights the importance of early guidance to minimise complications, pointing out **that "prevention is better than cure".**

It is important to instruct kidney patients about diet, treatment modality, comorbidities, prevention measures and complication control. It is essential that health education involves the team that cares for the individual. This was emphasised by the participants in the survey, who suggested that the nutritionist and the entire multi-professional team should be involved in providing guidance. This is in line with the study by Saxena and Rizk (2014), who mention that interdisciplinary work is effective when those responsible for providing guidance are trained to do so and can empower patients, making them responsible and co-responsible for improving their quality of life.

It's also important to remember that you have to look for an education strategy that can catch people's attention and arouse interest. Few professionals considered the structure of the PTE (as a pamphlet) to be of low applicability because reading documents doesn't appeal to many patients. For this reason, the intention arose to produce a booklet containing information about the disease, treatment, legislation, guidelines, as well as functioning as an instrument for identifying the individual and monitoring that helps treatment by the patient and the professional who attends to them.

It should be noted that even though there have been so many studies and research carried out on education with kidney patients, Greer, Crews and Boulware (2012) highlight the difficulties presented by professionals in carrying out educational activities with chronic kidney patients. These include: low awareness among individuals and low recognition of CKD as a medical problem; different views on CKD from primary care providers; lack of knowledge or adequate skills to educate people about CKD on the part of care providers; fear of the individual's (emotional) reaction; limitations on the time spent visiting the patient and lack of educational resources. Some of these aspects were also highlighted by the PTE analyses, where the professionals stressed that it is a technology that does not require a lot of time to be used, and does not bore the patient or the professional. After the changes made, which resulted in the booklet, this advantage was reinforced, since the individual is the owner of the tool, so it allows them to find out more or clarify doubts at any time.

Pagels, Hylander and Alvarsson (2015) developed a multidimensional support programme to be worked on with diabetic people that allows goals to be set and the individual's performance to be monitored with *feedback,* and showed positive results in terms of changes in health behaviour. This study reminds us of the need for teamwork to improve care for people with any pathology, as multidisciplinary care favours addressing all aspects involved in health and improving the individual's quality of life. This approach was also highlighted by the professionals who evaluated the TPP, recommending the participation of the nutritionist in the education of kidney patients, since nutritional guidance should be provided on an individual basis.

Ladin and Weiner (2015) presented a study carried out in dialysis centres in the United Kingdom and identified significant changes in the interpretation of information about possible treatments for chronic kidney disease, concluding that, depending on how the issues are addressed, individuals can make different decisions about the choice of treatment.

The way in which the information was approached was also highlighted by the professionals who evaluated the PTE, where the majority suggested including images to increase interest and make it easier for a larger group of people to understand, as well as changing the structure of the leaflet to something more interactive.

Skelton **et** *al.* (2015) highlight the insufficient number of kidney transplants for end-stage renal patients. This is why educating chronic kidney patients is of paramount importance. **However, the authors draw attention to the fact that an "information pack" is usually delivered to all** individuals, without taking into account their level of literacy, knowledge, beliefs, education, etc. They stress the importance of having a trained professional to provide individualised guidance.

The PTE evaluations showed that this technology can contribute to the prevention of complications resulting from CKD, with the potential for good results as it provides simple, practical and objective guidance on important topics that individuals should know.

Tuot et al. (2013) evaluated educational tools to be used with kidney patients and identified that educational materials are important in transmitting information, but that they must take into account the culture and level of knowledge of the individuals in order to have better results.

There are countless educational interventions used to work with CKD patients, but few use technology in their processes. Heiden et al. (2013) presented a prototype of a technology to help with the diet of chronic kidney disease patients which, according to the authors, still needs modifications and validation, but which seeks to give the individual the opportunity to be responsible for caring for their diet on a daily basis based on the guidance received from professionals.

Kennedy et al. (2014) presented a study carried out using focus groups with the aim of ensuring the participation of patients in generating information and using cartoons to generate very dynamic discussions.

It was suggested by the professionals that PTE should not only be applied to people treated in dialysis centres, but that it should be extended to outpatient clinics that treat individuals with kidney disease, so that primary prevention can be carried out early, avoiding complications resulting from CKD.

An educational website was designed to provide information on safety issues in chronic kidney disease. Participants were trained to use the site and then each received an identification number so that they could access it at any time and as many times as they felt necessary during the year. From then on, those responsible for the research had access to the number of times and the patient's search for the information, producing analyses that could or could not result in warning signs about the difficulty of understanding some topic on the part of that individual (DIAMANTIDIS, 2013).

Schatell (2013) presents various internet resources that can be used to support kidney patients, helping to provide information and answer questions. The following table summarises the main electronic addresses.

Chart 3 - Main electronic support tools for people with CKD

Electronic tool	Contribution
http://www.kidneyschool.org	Allows you to search for information on the subject at any time
http://www. aakp. org	Electronic health records
http://www.homedialysis.org	Information Sites
http://www.kidney.org	Information Sites
http://www.rsnhope.org	CKD advocacy websites
http://www.dialysispatients.org/about-dpc	CKD advocacy websites
http://www.hemodoc.com	Blogs with discussions on the subject
http://www.lindagromkomdkidneycare.blogspot.com	Blogs with discussions on the subject
http://homedialysis.org/webinars	Live webinars
http://www.pkdcure.org/learn/multimedia/webinars	Live webinars
Email groups and social networks	Sharing ideas and information

There are currently a number of follow-up recording tools provided by the SUS, such as the Pregnancy Card, which was created as a data recording tool to facilitate communication between prenatal care professionals and those who deliver babies, providing important pregnancy information for referrals and counter-referrals, as well as being a source of information for the Live Birth Information System (SINASC) (BRASIL, 2002). This tool needs to be filled in completely and clearly. It should always be with the pregnant woman, because if any complications occur, the professional who receives it will have enough information to provide the highest quality care possible.

Another example is the Child Health Handbook, which is an essential surveillance tool because it is the document that records the most important data and events regarding the child's health. It enables communication between the family, the professionals who care for the child and, above all, because it belongs to the child and the family and with them it passes through the different services and levels of care required in the exercise of health care.

Implemented in 2005 by the Ministry of Health, this booklet has undergone changes and records the child's identification, obstetric and neonatal history, diet, growth and development, use of iron and vitamin A supplements, oral, hearing and visual health, vaccinations, clinical complications, as well as guidelines for health promotion and the prevention of health problems such as accidents and domestic violence (BRASIL, 2005).

The Adolescent Health Booklet is available from the Ministry of Health's Virtual Health Library, in different versions for boys and girls (http://bvsms.saude.gov.br/bvs/publicacoes/caderneta saude adolescente menina.pdf and http://bvsms.saude.gov.br/bvs/publicacoes/caderneta saude adolescente menino.pdf)

It contains space to fill in personal details, information about adolescence, the adolescent's own responsibility in the process of self-discovery and self-care, a place to fill in the adolescent's personal preferences, blood type, illnesses, disabilities, medication in use, hospitalisations and surgeries already carried out, information about the Statute of the Child and Adolescent (ECA), health tips (including oral health and the odontogram), vaccination recommendations and records, information about changes identified at this stage of life, guidance on sexuality and protection against unwanted pregnancy and diseases transmitted through sexual relations.

There is also the Caderneta de Saúde da Pessoa Idosa (http://portalsaude. saude. gov.br/images/pdf/2015/julho/08/20-01-Miolo-Caderneta-vers-- ofinal2015.pdf), which was reformulated in 2014 and launched at the National Congress of Municipal Health Secretaries - CONASEMS, in June 2014, where important information about health conditions is recorded, helping health professionals to decide what actions are necessary for the elderly to have an active and healthy ageing. It allows health progress to be monitored and is highlighted as another action that reflects the commitment of all managers to the comprehensive health of the elderly population.

The booklet contains guidance on the rights of the elderly, the use and storage of medicines and access to them via the SUS, healthy eating, emphasising the need to carry it with you at all times, talking to the professionals who accompany you to clear up any doubts, the importance of physical activity, social inclusion in the community and relationships with the family, sexual orientation, identification data, medication in use according to medical prescription, notes on hospitalisations and surgeries performed, falls, allergies and vaccinations, appointment diary, anthropometric data and monitoring of blood pressure, glycaemia, weight and oral health, protocol for identifying vulnerable elderly people, environmental assessment, identification of chronic pain, as well as a place for additional information (http://portalsaude.saude.gov.br/index.php/o-ministerio/principal/secretarias/809-sas-raiz/daet- raiz/saude-da-pessoa-idosa/l2-saude-da-pessoa-idosa/12746-caderneta-de-saude-da-pessoa- idosa).

The Ministry of Health also provides the vaccination card for adolescents, adults, the elderly and the indigenous population, which serves only as a record of the vaccines administered and the scheduling of the next doses, as well as helping to prove vaccination during campaigns.

With regard to CKD patients undergoing dialysis, there is no specific tool for registering and monitoring these individuals. There is a **"booklet for kidney patients - health and citizenship"** available online (http://cartilhapacienterenal. cursoseconcursosnosite.com.br/?cat=3) which mainly covers information about the disease, important guidelines for treatment and laws that support CKD patients, but which does not allow for the monitoring of kidney patients through specific notes on their identification, treatment and general condition.

As there is no specific tool that can facilitate and improve the monitoring of CKD patients, this work **resulted in the "Renal Patient Handbook", which aims not only to provide** important

information and guidance to chronic kidney disease patients, but also to identify them as having the disease, making it easier to refer them to a specialised health unit if necessary, and above all, to provide important information in a clear and practical way that facilitates and assists in the treatment carried out by the professionals who treat these people in dialysis centres.

It should be noted that the suggestions and contributions of the participants who evaluated the TPP were of great value and relevance, highlighting that those involved are professionals with good experience in nephrology, with an average of 7.9 years working in the area. All have specific training in the area, strengthening the value of the considerations that favoured making the technology produced more comprehensive and full of important information when compared to the initial proposal of the work.

The booklet includes identification of the person, the professionals who accompany them, the dialysis centre where they are being treated, the person responsible (companion), the dialysis schedule, the medication being used, hepatitis immunisation control, guidance from the nutritionist, information about the disease, treatment, diet, healthy habits, the rights of the CKD patient who slips, as well as data recording each dialysis session with the date, duration and specific details of the procedure.

It is important to emphasise that the professionals taking part in this study evaluated the PTE, which was a tool initially produced with the intention of helping to prevent complications resulting from CKD. However, after analysis and contributions from the professionals, **the "Renal Patient Handbook"** was **produced, which** still needs to be tested in practice so that we can really conclude that the tool contributes to preventing complications and consequently improving the quality of life of these individuals.

6.1 Study limitations

We would like to highlight the limitations of this study. Initially, it was difficult to get the project approved by the Ethics Committee, which took a long time. Another setback was presenting the project to the directors of the clinics due to the difficulty of finding them available, a characteristic of their position. However, many professionals were very willing and filled in the evaluation form in good time. Others reported a lack of time and asked to be picked up at another time, which made it even more difficult.

CHAPTER 7

CONCLUSION

This study showed that professionals who work with people with CKD believe it is important to have technology to educate these individuals. Taking into account the opinion of these professionals, we made changes to the educational technology presented to them and proposed a tool for more detailed recording and monitoring of information about CKD patients.

The evaluation carried out by the nurses and doctors who accompany CKD patients in dialysis centres considered the technology proposed by this work to be feasible by the majority of interviewees who described it as easy, practical, objective and with accessible language.

The professionals believe that the technology has good applicability, including being able to be used in outpatient clinics, favouring primary and secondary prevention and helping to reduce the complications resulting from CKD.

It can be concluded that, through good health education strategies, people with CKD become better acquainted with their disease and the conditions that favour or disfavour their state of health. Thus, they feel responsible for their wellbeing, seeking to follow the guidelines provided by professionals and preventing the manifestations of complications, progression and worsening of their illness.

The result of this work was the creation of a tool to better record information related to the treatment of CKD patients, allowing them to be better monitored at all appointments, facilitating knowledge of the individual's state of health on the part of the entire team that assists them and making it possible to identify them as having a chronic disease that requires special care.

It's important to emphasise that the aim of the booklet is to help monitor kidney patients, but it doesn't exclude the need for guidance that must be provided by all the professionals involved in their care, as well as clarifying any doubts that may arise as the person becomes better acquainted with their condition.

This work also emphasises that the treatment and monitoring of CKD patients should be carried out by a multi-professional team, where each category has important functions, but one complements the other and all together offer the individual comprehensive care.

REFERENCES

ALVES, V. S. Um modelo de educação em saúde para o Programa Saúde da Família: pela integralidade da atenção e reorientação do modelo assistencial. **Comunic, Saúde, Educ,** v. 9, n.16, p.39-52, 2005.

ARAÚJO, M. H. A. et al. Investigation of urinary abnormalities and risk factors for kidney disease in the World Kidney Day campaigns in Northeast Brazil. **Rev Assoc Med Bras**, v. 60, n.5, p. 479-483, 2014.

BARBOSA. D. A. et al. Co-morbidity and mortality of patients starting dialysis. **Acta Paul Enferm.**, v.16, n.3, p.304-309, 2006.

BARRETO, M. S.; SILVA, M.A.A; SEZEREMETA, D.C.; BASÍLIO, G.; MARCON, S.S. Health knowledge and difficulties experienced in caring: perspective of family members of patients undergoing dialysis treatment. **Cienc Cuid Saude**, v.10, n.4, p.722-730, 2011.

BASTOS, M. G; KIRSZTAJN, G. M. Chronic kidney disease: importance of early diagnosis, immediate referral and structured interdisciplinary approach to improve outcome in patients not yet undergoing dialysis. **J Bras Nefrol**, v.33, n.1, p.93-108, 2011.

BRAGA, S. F. M. **Avaliação da Qualidade de Vida de Pacientes Idosos em Hemodiálise em Belo Horizonte - MG** - Belo Horizonte, 2009.

BRAZIL. Ministry of Health. Women's Health Technical Area. Secretariat for Health Policies. Prenatal and Birth Humanisation Programme. **Rev. Bras. Saúde Materninfant**, v. 2, p.69-71, 2002.

BRAZIL. Department of Strategic Programmatic Actions, Secretariat of Health Care, Ministry of Health. **Manual for the use of the child health booklet**. Brasília: Ministry of Health; 2005.

Ministry of Health. Health Surveillance Secretariat. Department of Health Situation Analysis. **Strategic action plan for tackling chronic non-communicable diseases (NCDs) in Brazil 2011-2022**, Brasilia: Ministry of Health, 2011.

Ministry of Health. Health Care Secretariat. Department of Specialised and Thematic Care. **Clinical Guidelines for the Care of Patients with Chronic Kidney Disease - CKD in the Unified Health System / Ministry of Health**. Department of Specialised and Thematic Care. Department of Specialised and Thematic Care. - Brasília: Ministry of Health, 2014.

BREITSAMETER, G.; THOMÉ, E. G. R.; SILVEIRA, D. T. Complications that lead chronic kidney patients to an emergency service. **Rev Gaúcha Enferm.**, v. 29, n.4, p. 543550, 2008.

BROGDON, R. M. A self-care educational intervention to improve knowledge of dietary phosphorus control in patients requiring haemodialysis: A pilot study. **Nephrology Nursing Journal**, v.40, n.4, p.

313-318, 2013.

CALDEIRA et al. Educational strategies to reduce serum phosphorus in hyperphosphatemic patients with chronic kidney disease: systematic review with meta-analysis. **Journal of Renal Nutrition**, v. 21, n. 4, p. 285-294, 2011.

CARNEIRO, R. F. **Proposal for educational technology to prevent the risk of hypertension in pregnancy: a collective construction**. 2014. 122 f. Dissertation (Master's in Collective Health) - University of Fortaleza, Fortaleza.

CARVALHO, S. R.; GASTALDO, D. Health promotion and empowerment: a reflection from critical-social post-structuralist perspectives. **Ciência & Saúde Coletiva**, v. 13, sup. 2, p. 2029-2040, 2008.

CARVALHO, C. A; SANTOS, F. R. Prevention and health promotion work with kidney patients cared for by an interdisciplinary team: challenges and constructions. **Rev. APS**, v. 12. n.3, p. 311-317, 2009.

CESARINO, C. B.; CASAGRANDE, L. D. R. Patient with chronic renal failure undergoing haemodialysis treatment: nurses' educational activity. **Rev. latino-am. Enfermagem**, v. 6, n. 4, p. 31-40, 1998.

CHOE, E.S.; LEE, J. Effects of a Face-to-face Self-management Programme on Knowledge, Self-care Practice and Kidney Function in Patients with Chronic Kidney Disease before the Renal Replacement Therapy. **J Korean Acad Nurs**, v. 42, n. 7, p. 1070-1078, 2012.

CLARKSON, K.A. Life on dialysis: A lived experience. **Nephrology Nursing Journal**, v. 71, n.1, p. 29-35, 2010.

COELHO, A.; DINIZ, A.; HARTZ, Z.; DUSSAULT, G. Integrated management of chronic kidney disease: analysis of an innovative policy in Portugal. **Rev por saúde pública**, v. 21, n.1, p. 69-79, 2014.

DIAMANTIDIS, C.J. Directed Use of the Internet for Health Information by Patients With Chronic Kidney Disease: Prospective Cohort Study. **J Med Internet Res**, v. 15, n.11, p. 251, 2013.

FAVÉ et al. Freins à la participation des patientes en stade 3 de la maladie rénale chronique à l'éducation thérapeutique porposée emréseau de santé. **Néphrologie & Thérapeutique**, v. 10, p. 112-117, 2014.

FORTES, V.L.F.; BETTINELLI, L.A.; POMATTI, D.M.; BROCK, J.; DOBNER, T. The journey of chronic kidney disease: from forewarning to discovery. **Rev Rene**, v. 14, n.3, p. 531540, 2013.

FREITAS, P.S. et al. Education in the prevention of chronic renal failure: the health team's view. IX International Congress of Education, Research and Management, 2011.

GREER, R.C.; CREWS, D.C.; BOULWARE, L.E. Challenges perceived by primary care providers to educating patients about chronic kidney disease. **Journal of Renal Care**, v. 38, n. 4, p. 174-181, 2012.

GRICIO, T.C.; KUSUMOTA, L.; CANDIDO, M.L. Perceptions and knowledge of patients with Chronic Kidney Disease undergoing conservative treatment. **Rev. Eletr. Enf.** [Internet], v.11, n. 4, p. 884-893, 2009.

GUBERT et *al.* Educational technologies in the school context: health education strategy in a public school in Fortaleza-CE. **Rev. Eletr. Enf**, v. 11, n. 1, p. 165-172, 2009.

GUIMARAES, R. Translational research: an interpretation. **Ciênc Saúde Coletiva**, v. 18, p. 1731-1744, 2013.

HEIDEN, S. et al. A Diet Management Information and Communication System to Help Chronic Kidney Patients Cope with Diet Restrictions. **MEDINFO**, p. 543-547, 2013.

HUANG, X.; CARRERO, J.J. Better prevention than cure: optimal patient preparation for renal replacement therapy. **Kidney International**, v. 85, p. 507-510, 2014.

JACOPETTI, A. Social and communication practices of kidney patients on the Facebbok of the Pro-Rim Foundation. **Rev. Estud. Comun.**,v. 12, n. 27, p. 81-89, 2011.

JUNIOR, J.E.R. Chronic Kidney Disease: Definition, Epidemiology and Classification. **J. Bras. Nefrol.**, v. 26, n. 3, p. 1-3, 2004.

KARAVETIAN, M.; VRIES, N.; RIZK, R., ELZEIN, H. Dietary educational interventions for management of hyperphosphatemia in haemodialysis patients: a systematic review and meta-analysis. **Nutrition Reviews**, v. 72, n. 7, p. 471-482, 2014.

KENNEDY, A. Developing cartoons for long-term condition self-management information. **BMC Health Services Research**, v. 14, p. 60, 2014.

K/DOQI. Clinical Practice Guidelines For Chronic Kidney Disease: Evaluation, Classification and Stratification. **Am J Kidney Dis**, v. 39, 2002.

LADIN, K.; WEINER, D.E. Better informing older patients with kidney failure in an era of patient-centred care. **Am J Kidney Dis**, v. 65, n. 3, p. 372-374, 2015.

LEWIS, A.L., STABLER, K.A., WELCH, J.L. Perceived informational needs, problems, or concerns among patients with Stage 4 chronic kidney disease. **Nephrology Nursing Journal**, v. 37, n. 2, p. 143-149, 2010.

MAGALHÃES, J. L. F; SANTOS, Z. M. S. A. **Lifestyle of elderly hypertensive patients: analysing the impact of a health education technology.** Master's dissertation, University of Fortaleza - UNIFOR, 2009, 61 f.

L'orientamento del paziente uremico nella scelta del tratamento sostitutivo: ruolo dell'ambulatório di predialisi. **G Ital Nefrol**, v. 29, n. 5, p. 592-598, 2012.

MARTINS, M.R.I; CESARINO, C.B. Update on education and rehabilitation programmes for chronic kidney patients undergoing haemodialysis. **J Bras Nefrol.**, v. 26, n. 1, p. 45-50, 2004.

MENDES, E. V. **Health Care Networks**. Brasília, DF: PAHO, 2011.

MERHY, E.E. In search of tools to analyse health technologies: information and daily life in a service, questioning and managing health work. In: MERHY, E.E.; ONOKO, R. organisers. **Acting in Health: a challenge for the public**. 2 ed.: Hucitec, São Paulo: 2002.

MORANTE, J.J.H. et *al*. Effectiveness of a Nutrition Education Programme for the Prevention and Treatment of Malnutrition in End-Stage Renal Disease. **Journal of Renal Nutrition**, v. 24, n. 1, p. 42-49, 2014.

MURPHY F. et al. Patient management in chronic kidney disease stages 4 to 5. **Journal of Renal Care**, v. 34, n. 4, p. 191-198, 2008.

NASCIMENTO, C.D.; MARQUES, I.R. Nursing interventions in the most frequent complications during the haemodialysis session: a literature review. **Rev Bras Enferm.**, v. 58, n. 6, p. 719-722, 2005.

NOZAKI, C., OKA, M., CHABOYER, W. The effects of a cognitive behavioural therapy programme for self-care on haemodialysis patients. **International Journal of Nursing Practice**, v. 11, p. 228-236, 2005.

NUNES, J.A.W. Education of Patients With Chronic Kidney Disease at the Interface of Primary Care Providers and Nephrologists **Advances in Chronic Kidney Disease**, v. 20, n. 4, p. 370-378, 2013.

PAES-BARRETO, J.G. et al. Can Renal Nutrition Education Improve Adherence to a Low- Protein Diet in Patients With Stages 3 to 5 Chronic Kidney Disease? **Journal of Renal Nutrition**, v. 23, n. 3, p. 164-171, 2013.

PAGELS, A.A.; HYLANDER, B.; ALVARSSON, M. A multi-dimensional support programme for patients with diabetic kidney disease. **Journal of Renal Care**, v. 41, n. 3, p. 187-194, 2015.

PERES, L. A. B. et. *al.* Epidemiological study of end-stage renal disease in western Paraná. An experience of 878 cases treated over 25 years. **J Bras Nefrol**, v. 32, n.1, p. 5156, 2010.

POLIT, D. F.; BECK, C. T.; HUNGLER, B. P. **Fundamentals of nursing research: methods, evaluation and utilisation.** 5. ed. Porto Alegre: Artmed, 2004.

PORTER, E.; WATSON, D.; BARGMAN, J.M. Education for Patients With Progressive CKD and Acute-Start Dialysis. **Advances in Chronic Kidney Disease**, v. 20, n. 4, p. 302-310, 2013.

PROSCIA, A. MyPlate for Healthy Eating With Chronic Kidney Disease (MyPlate Education for Patients With Chronic Kidney Disease Receiving Haemodialysis and Peritoneal Dialysis Treatment) **Journal of Renal Nutrition**, v. 24, n. 3, p. 23-25, 2014.

QUEIROZ, M.V.O.; DANTAS, M.C.Q.; RAMOS, I.C.; JORGE, M.S.B. Tecnologia do cuidado ao paciente renal crônico: enfoque educativo-terapêutico a partir das necessidades dos sujeitos. **Texto Contexto Enferm**, v. 17, n. 1, p. 55-63, 2008.

RAMOS, I. C.; QUEIROZ, M. V. O.; JORGE, M. S. B. Care in a situation of Chronic Kidney Disease: social representations elaborated by adolescents. **Revista Brasileira de Enfermagem**, v. 61, n. 2, p. 193-200, 2008.

RIELLA, M.C. **Princípios de Nefrologia e distúrbios hidroeletrolíticos.** 5 ed. Rio de Janeiro: Guanabara Koogan, 2010.

RIOUX et al. Effect of an in-hospital chronic kidney disease education programme among patients with unplanned urgent-start dialysis. **Clinical Journal of the American Society of Nephrology**, v. 6, p. 799-804, 2011.

ROCHA, P.K. et *al.* Care and technology: approach through the care model. **Rev Bras Enferm**, v. 6, n. 1, p. 113-115, 2008.

ROCHA, R.P.F. **Necessidades de orientação de enfermagem para o autocuidado visando a qualidade de vida de clientes em terapia de hemodiálise**. Master's dissertation, Rio de Janeiro State University,

2010.

RODRIGUEZ, C.R. et al. Recovering activity and illusion: the nephrology medical day hospital. **Nefrologia**, v. 31, n. 5, p. 545-559, 2011.

ROSOL, C.C.; BEUTER, M.; BRONDANI, C.M.; TIMM, A.M.B.; PAULETTO, M.R.; CORDEIRO, F.R. Self-care of renal patients under conservative treatment: an integrative review. **R. pesq.: cuid. Fundam.**, v. 5, n. 5, p. 102-110, 2013.

SALLY, H.; BREN, V. Essential Components of an Infection Prevention Programme for Outpatient Hemodialysis Centres. **Seminars in Dialysis**, v. 26, n. 4, p. 384-398, 2013.

SANCHO, L.G; DAIN, D. Analysing cost-effectiveness in relation to renal replacement therapies: how to think about studies in relation to these interventions in Brazil? **Cad. Saúde Pública**, v. 24, n. 6, p. 1279-1290, 2008.

SANTOS, Z.M.S.Z.; LIMA, H.P. Educational technology in health in the prevention of hypertension in workers: analysis of changes in lifestyle. **Texto Contexto Enferm**, Florianópolis, v. 17, n. 1, p. 90-97, 2008.

SANTOS, I.; ROCHA, R.P.F.; BERARDINELLI, L.M.M. Necessidades de orientação de enfermagem para o autocuidado de clientes em terapia de hemodiálise. **Rev Bras Enferm**, v. 64, n. 2, p. 335-342, 2011.

SARDENBERG, C.; SOUSA, N.K.G; CENDOROGLO, M.N; CANZIANI, M.E.F. **Doença Renal Crônica: Diagnóstico e Tratamento.** v.3. Barueri, São Paulo: Manole, 2007.

SAXENA, N.; RIZK, D. V. The interdisciplinary team: the whole is larger than the parts. **Advances in Chronic Kidney Disease**, v. 21, n. 4, p. 333-337, 2014.

SESSO et al. Brazilian Chronic Dialysis Survey 2013 - Analysis of trends between 2011 and 2013. **J Bras Nefrol.**, v. 36, n. 4, p. 476-481, 2014.

SCHATELL, D. Web-based kidney education: supporting patient self-management. **Seminars in Dialysis**, v. 26, n. 2, p. 154-158, 2013.

SILVA, C.K.P. Adherence of patients with chronic renal failure to dialysis therapy. Recife-PE, 2012.

SILVA, L.K.; BREGMAN, R.; LESSI, D.; LEIMANN, B. Mariane Branco Alves Essay on blindness: mortality of patients with chronic kidney disease on emergency haemodialysis. **Ciência & Saúde**

Coletiva, v. 17, n. 11, p. 2971-2980, 2012.

SILVA, M.C.O.S., SILVA, K.L., SILVA, P.A.B. et al. The waiting room as a space for education and health promotion for people with chronic renal failure on haemodialysis. **J. res.: Fundam. Care,** v. 5, n. 3, p. 253-263, 2013.

SKELTON, S.L. et *al.* Applying best practices to designing patient education for patients with end-stage renal disease pursuing kidney transplant. **Prog Transplant,** v. 25, n. 1, p. 77-84, 2015.

SZUSTER et *al.* Survival of dialysis patients in SUS in Brazil. **Cad. Saúde Pública,** v. 28, n. 3, p. 415-424, 2012.

TAMURA et al. Educational programmes improve the preparation for dialysis and survival of patients with chronic kidney disease. **Kidney International,** v. 85, p. 686-692, 2014.

TRAVAGIM, D.S. A.; KUSUMOTA, L. The role of nurses in the prevention and progression of chronic kidney disease. **Rev. enferm**. UERJ, Rio de Janeiro, v. 17, n. 3, p. 388-393, 2009.

TUOT et al. Assessment of Printed Patient-Educational Materials for Chronic Kidney Disease. **Am J Nephrol,** v. 38, p. 184-194, 2013.

NEPHROLOGY UNIT OF THE HOSPITAL SAMARITANO DE SÃO PAULO. **General dietary guidelines for chronic renal patients**. São Paulo, 2010.

XIV LATINO AMERICAN SCIENTIFIC INITIATION MEETING AND X LATINO AMERICAN POST-GRADUATION MEETING, 2012, São José dos Campos, SP: Universidade do Vale do Paraíba. VASCONCELLOS, A.M.A.; BRAGA, E.C.L; SOAR, C. Effect of a nutritional programme on the control of hyperkalemia in patients with chronic renal failure, 2012.

Appendix 1

LETTER OF INVITATION

Dear Professional,

I am a student on the Master's programme in Collective Health at the University of Fortaleza - UNIFOR, and I am carrying out research entitled **PROPOSAL FOR EDUCATIONAL TECHNOLOGY IN THE PREVENTION OF COMPLICATIONS ARISING FROM CHRONIC KIDNEY DISEASE, with the** aim of *constructing and validating an educational technology for the prevention and/or control of the risk of complications arising from Chronic Kidney Disease.* To ensure the success of this research, I would like to ask you to take part in the evaluation of the

Educational Technology Proposal (ETP) and to answer the **ETP Evaluation Questionnaire.**

I would like to emphasise that your participation is voluntary, in accordance with Resolution 466/2012 of the National Research Ethics Committee (CONEP/CNS/MS). If you agree to contribute to this study, please sign the attached Informed Consent Form (ICF).

I would like to stress that the results of this research could make it possible to add new strategies that are favourable to the quality of life of patients with Chronic Kidney Disease by (re)planning actions in Haemodialysis Centres, with a view to preventing complications and/or controlling Chronic Kidney Disease, with effective and efficient implementation of care.

I'm sure I can count on your contribution and thank you in advance for your attention.

Yours sincerely,

Maria Cecilia Cavalcante Barreira
Researcher

Appendix 2

INFORMED CONSENT FORM

RESEARCH TITLE: PROPOSAL FOR EDUCATIONAL TECHNOLOGY TO PREVENT COMPLICATIONS FROM CHRONIC KIDNEY DISEASE

RESPONSIBLE RESEARCHER: Maria Cecilia Cavalcante Barreira

PARTICIPATION IN THE RESEARCH:

Dear Employee,

I would like to ask you to take part in this research and answer the questionnaire, which contains questions related to the general objective of the research - to *build and validate an educational technology for the prevention and/or control of complications resulting from Chronic Kidney Disease.*

I would like to point out that your participation will be extremely important for the development of the research and for the application of the results, which will make it possible for Dialysis Clinic Professionals to reflect on them, as well as being an instrument for recording data on the care of chronic kidney patients and could also be used as a proposal for educational technology (PTE) with the aim of promoting health through the prevention and/or control of risk factors for complications arising from Chronic Kidney Disease.

I would like to make it clear that the information collected will only be used for the purposes of the research, and that you are free to withdraw from the research at any time, even after you have started the interview. I would also like to make it clear that your anonymity will be preserved and that you will not be harmed in any way.

RISKS AND DISCOMFORTS

The study poses no risk to their physical or emotional integrity, nor to the services offered by these institutions.

BENEFITS

I would emphasise that the results of the study will make it possible to (re)plan the health actions carried out by professionals at dialysis clinics, with a view to promoting health with an emphasis on preventing complications and controlling Chronic Kidney Disease, through the effective and efficient implementation of care.

FORMS OF ASSISTANCE

If you need any advice or have any questions about the research, you can contact the researcher responsible, Maria Cecilia Cavalcante Barreira, on (85) 8563-0333.

CONFIDENTIALITY

All the information you give me will only be used for this research. Your answers will remain secret and your name will not appear anywhere in the interview, nor when the results are publicised.

CLARIFICATIONS

If you have any questions about the research and/or the methods used in it, you can contact the researcher responsible at any time.

Researcher responsible Address: Maria Cecilia Cavalcante Barreira Contact telephone number: (85) 8563-0333 Opening hours: 2^a to 6^a - 08:00 to 12:00 and 14:00 to 18:00.

If you wish to obtain information about your rights and the ethical aspects involved in the research, you can consult the Ethics Committee of the University of Fortaleza, in Fortaleza-CE.

REIMBURSEMENT OF EXPENSES:

If you agree to take part in the research, you will not receive any financial compensation.

AGREEMENT TO PARTICIPATE:

If you agree to take part, you must fill in and sign the Post-Inclarified Consent Form below, and you will receive a copy of this form.

The **research participant** or their legal representative, if applicable, must initial all the pages of the Informed Consent Form - affixing their signature on the last page of the Form.

The **researcher responsible** must also initial all the pages of the Informed Consent Form - affixing their signature to the last page of the form.

POST INFORMED CONSENT

By this instrument, which fulfils the legal requirements, you.

____ ,

bearer of an identity card, declares that, after reading the Informed Consent Form in detail, he/she has had the opportunity to ask questions, clarify doubts that have been duly explained by the researchers, is aware of the services and procedures to which he/she will be subjected and, having no doubts about what has been read and explained, signs his/her FREE AND INFORMED CONSENT to voluntarily participate in this research. And, in agreement, signs this form.

Fortaleza-Ce,de de.

____

Signature of research participant

____

Researcher's signature

Human Research Ethics Committee University of Fortaleza. Av. Washington Soares, 1321, Bloco da Reitoria, Sala da Vice-Reitoria de Pesquisa e Pós-Graduação, 1° andar. Edson Queiroz neighbourhood, CEP 6081-905. Telephone (85) 3477-3122. Fortaleza-CE

Appendix 3
Educational Technology Proposal (ETP) - Prevention of complications arising from Chronic Kidney Disease

PREVENTIVE AND/OR CONTROL MEASURES FOR COMPLICATIONS RESULTING FROM CHRONIC KIDNEY DISEASE
Nutrition
Adequate salt and sugar intake
Avoid sausages and tinned foods
Avoid foods high in sugar
Take the salt shaker off the table
Reduce the amount of salt in food preparation
Use natural spices (garlic, onion, chives, bay leaves, basil, oregano, pepper, parsley,

vinegar, etc.).
Fluid intake
Control intake of water, coffee, soft drinks, tea, milk, broths and soups
Protein intake
Choose meat, chicken, fish or eggs for lunch and dinner (in adequate quantities)
Vegetable fat intake
Favour vegetable cream, margarine or unsalted butter
Potassium intake
Cook vegetables (cauliflower, spinach, aubergine, green beans, okra, broccoli, courgettes, potatoes, cassava and pumpkin) in water and discard the cooking water.
Preference for vegetables
Give preference to fruit and vegetables Do not eat star fruit or drink its natural juice
Blood pressure and glycaemic control
Blood pressure
Measure blood pressure weekly
Blood sugar
Carry out periodic examinations according to medical advice
Habits
Smoking
Avoid using cigarettes and other drugs (cannabis, crack, cocaine)
Alcoholism
Avoid drinking alcoholic beverages
Regular physical exercise
Exercise according to medical advice and guidance
Adequate sleep and rest
Sleep (08 to 10 hours a night) Rest (02 to 03 hours a day)
Stress management
Search for leisure options Look for social support that helps reduce stress (groups, associations) Follow spiritual guidance that you believe in and that brings relief from anxieties and fears.
Systematic attendance at appointments
Always be present at scheduled appointments (medical or nursing) and haemodialysis sessions
Medication
Risk of self-medication
Use only prescribed medication
Regular use of prescribed medication (if applicable)
Take the medicine exactly as prescribed
Dialysis

Knowledge of the procedure
Clarify doubts about dialysis whenever they arise
Transplant
Seek information on the indications for transplantation and precautions to avoid the need for this procedure

Appendix 4

PTE VALIDATION QUESTIONNAIRE

Nurse ( ) Doctor ( )

1. Identification Data
1   Age (years) 2 Sex

3   Years of: Training (years) Professional practice (years)

---

4   Postgraduate studies.

4.1 Specialisation ( ) Area _______________________________________

4.2 Residence ( ) Area ____

4.3 Master's Degree ( ) Area ____________________________________

4.4 Doctorate ( ) Area ____

5   Length of service at:

Specialised Nephrology Care

II. Educational Technology Proposal (ETP)

1.   In your opinion, what is the feasibility/applicability of the ETP?

____

____

____

2.   Does the TPP cover all the preventive measures and/or control of the risk factors for complications of Chronic Kidney Disease?

Yes ( ) Justify ____

No ( ) Justify ____

---

3.   What would you change or add to the TPP in relation to:

a) Scope

____

____

____

b) content

____

____

____

c) Objectivity

____

____

____

d) Structure

____

____

____

e) language

____

____

____

4. PTE can contribute to preventing and/or controlling the risk of complications from Chronic Kidney Disease:

a) Professional who accompanies the kidney patient?
Yes ( ) Justify

____

____

No ( ) Justify

____

____

____

b) Renal patient?
Yes ( ) Justify

____

____

No ( ) Justify

5. What suggestions would you make to help improve the ETP?

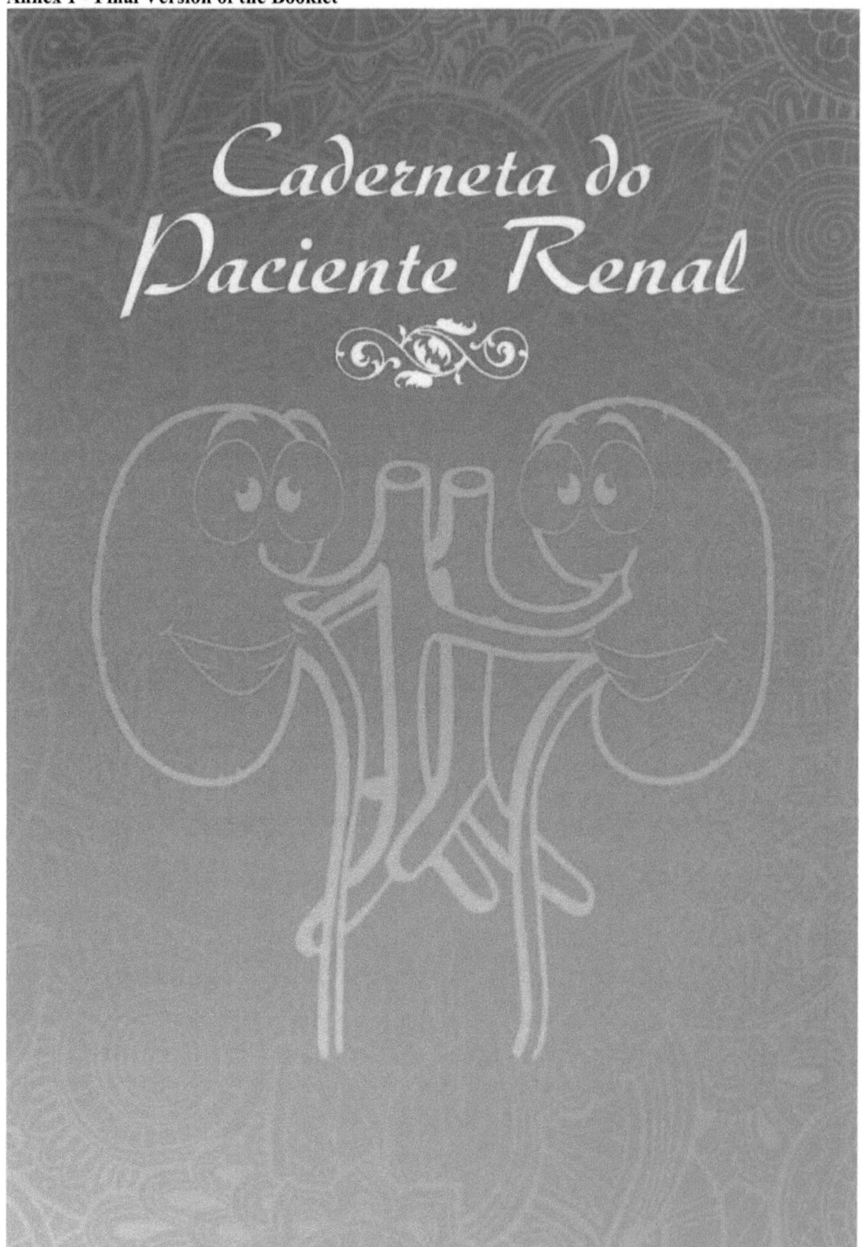
Caderneta do
Paciente Renal

Identificação

Nome:_______________________________
Data de Nascimento:___________ Idade: _____
Sexo:_______________________________
CPF: _______________________________
RG:______________ Órgão emissor: ______

Tipo sanguíneo:___________ Fator Rh:_______

Estado Civil: ____________ Filhos: _________
Naturalidade: _______________________
Nacionalidade: ______________________
Endereço: ___________________________
Cidade:________________ Estado:________
Ocupação: __________________________
Telefone: ___________________________
Email:______________________________

Em situação de emergência, contatar:
Nome:_______________________________
Telefone:____________________________
Parentesco:__________________________

Doença de base:______________________
Início da diálise:______________________
Convênio:____________________________
Unidade de Saúde em que realiza Hemodiálise:
____
Endereço:____________________________
Telefone: ___________________________
Profissionais responsáveis:
____
____
____

( ) Hemodiálise   ( ) DPI   ( ) CAPD

Calendário de diálise semanal

DIA/HORÁRIO	SEG	TER	QUA	QUI	SEX	SAB

Medicamentos em uso:

Medicamento	Prescrição

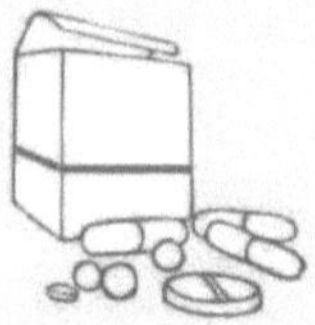

Tipo de acesso:
( ) cateter   ( ) fístula arteriovenosa
Local:

Observações relativas ao acesso vascular

____
____
____
____

Controle de Imunização contra Hepatite B:

Doses	1º dose	2º dose	3º dose	Reforço
Data				
Anti-HBS				
Data		Valor		

Observações:

O Ministério da Saúde diz que as doenças crônicas são as principais causas de mortes no mundo, causando perda da qualidade de vida e impacto econômico para a sociedade em geral.

A Doença Renal Crônica (DRC) é um problema de saúde pública em todo o mundo e o número de pacientes que precisam de acompanhamento para tratá-la vem aumentando bastante.

Em 2013 no Brasil o número total estimado de pacientes em diálise foi de 100.397 e vem aumentando ao longo dos anos: em 2012 eram 97.586, 91.314 em 2011, e 54.523 em 2003. Os que iniciaram tratamento foram 34.161.

É preciso ter hábitos saudáveis que ajudem a prevenir a DRC e suas complicações. Mas se a doença for descoberta e estiver no início, o tratamento será melhor direcionado e pode atrasar a evolução da doença em muitos anos.

Diante do grande problema que a doença tem se tornado para a população brasileira e com a intenção de ajudar e apoiar os portadores de DRC, essa Caderneta é uma proposta de ferramenta para registrar as informações relacionadas ao tratamento e acompanhamento do paciente em todas as consultas e facilitar o conhecimento desse paciente por parte da equipe de saúde que o acompanha.

O QUE É A DOENÇA RENAL CRÔNICA (DRC)

A DRC é uma doença irreversível que faz com que os rins não realizem mais sua função. A principal função dos rins é filtrar o sangue e eliminar as substâncias tóxicas que fazem mal ao organismo.

É uma doença lenta e no início não causa sintomas fáceis de perceber. Mas à medida que evolui, como o rim fica incapaz de filtrar o sangue e expulsar as substâncias tóxicas, pode causar enjoos, vômitos, pressão alta, inchaço e anemia.

Algumas pessoas podem ter o risco maior de apresentar a DRC:
a) Pessoas com diabetes;
b) Pessoas com pressão alta;
c) Idosos;
d) Obesos;
e) Pessoas com história de doenças do coração, e acidente vascular cerebral (AVC);
f) Pessoas com DRC na família (parentes);
g) Fumantes.

COMO TRATAR?

O tratamento da DRC depende do grau da doença e começa com medicamentos e dieta. Em muitos casos, é preciso outro tratamento que substitua a função dos rins que podem ser: diálise peritoneal, hemodiálise e transplante renal.

A diálise peritoneal usa parte de uma membrana do abdome (peritônio) para filtrar o sangue. Essa modalidade de tratamento remove substâncias tóxicas acumuladas no sangue como ureia, creatinina, potássio, fosfato e água para a solução de diálise (dialisato), que é introduzida no abdome e a membrana peritoneal acaba funcionando como o capilar da hemodiálise, regulando a troca de água e solutos.

A hemodiálise é o processo de filtragem do sangue (quando os rins do paciente não o conseguem fazer) de substâncias que precisam ser retiradas da corrente sanguínea através de uma máquina. Normalmente acontece 3 vezes por semana com duração de 4 horas em média. Em alguns casos, durante as sessões, as pessoas podem sentir: queda da pressão, câimbras, enjoos, vômitos, dor de cabeça, dor no peito, dor nas costas, coceira, febre e calafrio.

O transplante é a substituição do rim doente por um rim saudável vindo de um doador (vivo ou morto). Quando o médico avalia o paciente e diz que ele precisa de um transplante, reunem-se os documentos, que vão ser avaliados por uma equipe e então o paciente entra na fila do transplante. A fila não é organizada por tempo de espera e sim pela compatibilidade entre doador e receptor, além da urgência do transplante. Se houver empate, o tempo de espera pode ser considerado para desempate, entre outras características.

Sal e açúcar

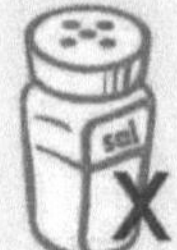

- Evitar linguiça, salsicha, enlatados
- Evitar alimentos ricos em açúcar
- Tirar o saleiro da mesa
- Reduzir a quantidade de sal no preparo dos alimentos
- Usar temperos naturais (alho, cebola, cebolinha, louro, manjericão, orégano, pimenta, salsa, vinagre etc.)

Líquidos

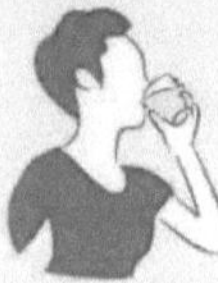

- Controlar a quantidade de água, café, refrigerante, chá, leite, caldos e sopas.

Proteínas

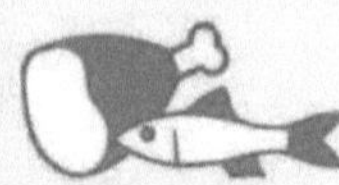

- Escolher carne, frango, peixe ou ovo na refeição do almoço e do jantar (em quantidade adequada).

Gordura vegetal

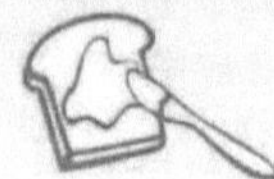

- Preferir creme vegetal, margarina ou manteiga sem sal

Potássio

- Cozinhar couve-flor, espinafre, berinjela, vagem, quiabo, brócolis, abobrinha, batata, mandioquinha e abóbora em água e descartar a água do cozimento

Preferir vegetais

- Dar preferência para frutas e verduras. Não comer carambola nem tomar o suco natural dessa fruta.

Pressão Arterial
- Medir a Pressão Arterial semanalmente

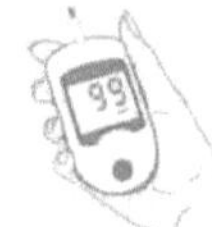

Glicemia
- Realizar exame de glicemia sempre que solicitado pelo médico/profissionais que acompanham

HÁBITO

Fumo
- Evitar uso de cigarro e outras drogas (maconha, crack, cocaína, entre outras).

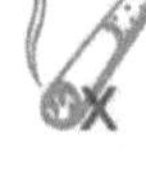

Álcool
- Evitar o consumo de bebidas alcoólicas.

Exercício físico
- Realizar exercício de acordo com indicação e orientação médica.

Sono e repouso
- Sono (08 a 10 horas por noite).
- Repouso (02 a 03 horas por dia).

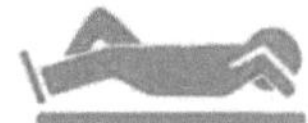

Cuidado com o estresse
- Buscar opções de lazer.
- Procurar apoio social (grupos, associações).
- Seguir orientações espirituais em que acredite e que tragam alívio das angústias e medos.
- Estar sempre presente nas consultas marcadas e sessões de hemodiálise.

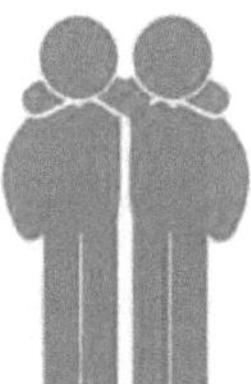

Automedicação
- Utilizar somente medicamentos prescrito.

Uso da medicação prescrita (se for caso)
- Tomar, conforme prescrição, o medicamento exatamente como foi orientado.

Tratamento
- Esclarecer dúvidas sobre a diálise sempre que surgirem.
- Buscar informações sobre as indicações de transplante e cuidados para evitar a necessidade deste procedimento.

Cuidados com acesso vascular

O cateter da hemodiálise é uma via de acesso vascular temporária, enquanto se espera o amadurecimento da fístula arteriovenosa. Portanto, são necessários cuidados para sua preservação e manutenção:

- Não molhe o curativo, se isto ocorrer, procure a unidade de diálise e peça para refazer o seu curativo. O curativo molhado pode propiciar infecção;
- Não dormir do lado do cateter;
- Não tracionar ou dobrar o cateter;
- Se o cateter apresentar sangramento, procure a unidade de diálise imediatamente;
- Não usar o cateter fora da unidade, somente profissionais capacitados podem ter acesso as vias do cateter.

Cuidados com a Fístula Arteriovenosa (FAV)

- Observar diariamente se a FAV está funcionando (se existe o tremor), colocando a mão sobre a cicatriz ou colocando o local da cicatriz sobre o ouvido (para ouvir o tremor); qualquer alteração percebida deve ser comunicada à equipe de enfermagem da diálise;
- Manter o local sempre limpo, lavando sempre com água e sabonete. Isto evita infecções que podem inutilizar a fístula. Qualquer sinal de inchaço e/ou vermelhidão deve ser comunicado imediatamente;
- Não usar roupas ou acessórios (relógios, pulseiras, entre outros) que apertem o braço da FAV;
-

- Não permitir que afiram pressão, apliquem medicações e coletem exames no braço da FAV.
- Não fazer força com o braço da FAV, ou movimentos tipo serrar, martelar, cortar lenha, usar furadeira, remar ou pescar.
- Não coçar e tirar as "casquinhas" das punções.
- Ao retirar as agulhas, ter paciência e esperar o tempo necessário para parar de sangrar, sem apertar demais – apertando demais, o fluxo de sangue na FAV pode parar, podendo fechar a FAV.
- Seis (6) horas depois de retiradas as agulhas, o curativo deve ser retirado. Se ainda continuar sangrando, fazer novo curativo e na próxima diálise avisar ao profissional que o acompanha.
- Medicações mais prejudiciais aos rins (nefrotóxicas): antiinflamatórios (principalmente os não esteroides: AINES), antibióticos, analgésicos, contrastes radiológicos.

Orientações do Nutricionista:

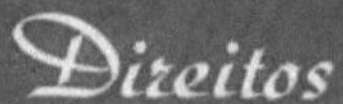

Direitos

LEIS QUE AMPARAM O PORTADOR DE DRC

Decreto Nº 7612 de 17 de novembro de 2011: Plano Nacional dos Direitos da Pessoa com Deficiência- Plano Viver sem Limite.

Portaria Nº 666 de 17 de julho de 2012: Protocolo Clínico e Diretrizes Terapêuticas – Imunosupressão no Transplante Renal.

Decreto Lei 5296 de 02 de dezembro de 2004: Lei da Acessibilidade.

Constituição Federal (artigo 196): "Saúde é direito de todos e dever do Estado"

Lei Nº 7853/89 e Decreto 3298 de 20 de dezembro de 1999: Apoio à pessoas portadoras de deficiência/ Política Nacional para a Integração da Pessoa Portadora de Deficiência.

Portaria 1168/GM de 15 de junho de 2004: regulamento técnico dos serviços de diálises.

Lei Nº 9434 de 04 de fevereiro de 1997 e Lei Nº 10211 de 23 de março de 2001: transplante de órgão/tecidos e tratamento.

Carta dos Direitos dos Usuários da Saúde

E SE EU NÃO PUDER TRABALHAR?

O paciente em programa de hemodiálise que é segurado pelo INSS (contribuiu por mais de 12 meses para a Previdência Social), pode dar entrada no Auxílio Doença. É preciso reunir alguns documentos e procurar o posto do INSS mais próximo à sua residência.

Se for confirmada invalidez, o segurado pode receber aposentadoria (após passar por perícia médica).

Portadores de insuficiência renal também têm direito a isenção do imposto de renda assegurado pela Lei Nº 8541 de 23 de dezembro de 1992 e instrução normativa Nº 49 de 10 de maio de 1999.

Em alguns casos o paciente também pode sacar o FGTS.

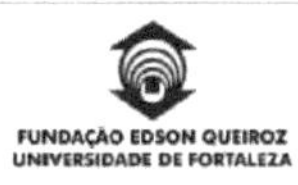

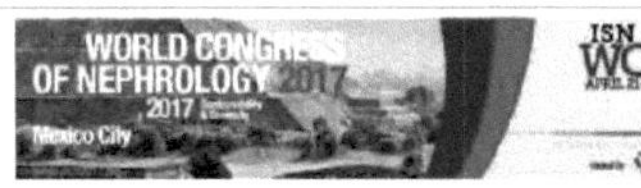

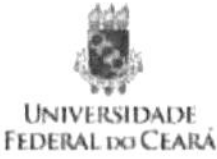

UNIVERSIDADE
FEDERAL DO CEARÁ

Construction and validation of an educational tool for the follow-up and prevention of complications of patients with chronic kidney disease

Maria Cecília Cavalcante Barreira[1], Danielle Teixeira Queiroz[2], Elizabeth De Francesco Daher[3], Geraldo Bezerra da Silva Junior[1]

[1]Public Health Graduate Program, Health Sciences Center, University of Fortaleza. Fortaleza, Ceará, Brazil;
[2]Nursing School, Health Sciences Center, University of Fortaleza. Fortaleza, Ceará, Brazil.
[3]School of Medicine, Department of Internal Medicine, Federal University of Ceará. Fortaleza, Ceará, Brazil.

Background

Chronic kidney disease (CKD) is an increasing public health problem. In Brazil there are currently more than 111,000 patients in dialysis. It is extremely important to educate CKD patients about the disease itself, treatment and measures to slow CKD progression. The aim of this study is to describe the process of elaboration and validation of an educational tool to people with CKD.

Methods

This is a methodological study with descriptive nature to elaborate and validate an educational technology for CKD patients and a tool for registering information related to CKD treatment. The study was conducted in dialysis clinics in the city of Fortaleza, Ceará, Brazil, with participation of physicians and nurses working in these centers for at least 2 years. These workers were consulted to evaluate the proposed technology through a questionnaire assessing its viability and applicability.

Results

The assessed data points that 9 (75%) considered the technology possible to be applicable. The technology includes preventive measures for CKD, according to 8 of the interviewed (66.6%). For the majority of participants (75%), the technology has important contributions for the healthcare workers in preventing CKD complications. The majority of participants (83.3%) reported the great importance of the technology for the individuals as having CKD in the search for changing habits, adaptation to treatment and quality of life improvement. It was suggested an extension of the project for outpatients' clinics (to include people in conservative treatment) and not to restrict it to dialysis clinics. Some suggestions were made by the workers and it was taken into consideration to elaborate the tool for CKD people follow-up.

Chart 1. Educational Technology Proposal (PTE) - Prevention of Complications from Chronic Kidney Disease.

Results

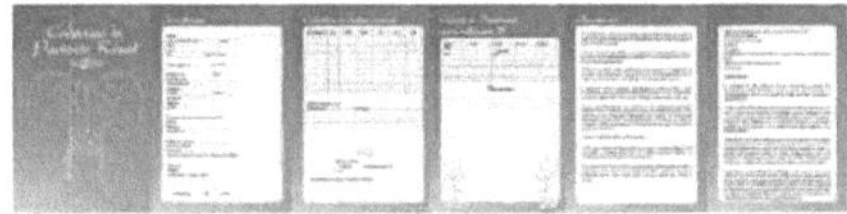

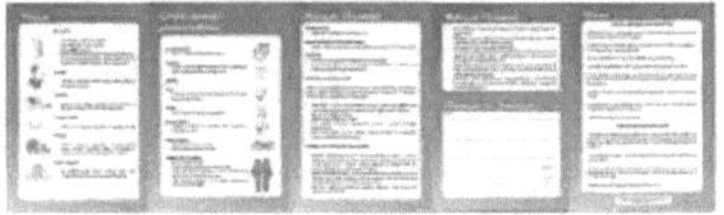

Conclusions

The creation of this tool aimed a more adequate registration of information related to CKD treatment and tries to allow a better follow-up of these individuals in all consultations, facilitating the identification of their health conditions by the healthcare team and allowing the identification of these individuals as having CKD and, consequently, needing special care. This tool also will serve as educational tool, giving patients basic information about CKD.

References

1. Queiroz MV, Dantas MC, Ramos IC, Jorge MS. Care technology for the chronic renal disease patient: educational-therapeutic focus from the subject's needs. *Texto Contexto Enferm* 2008; 17: 55-63.
2. Santos I, Rocha RPF. Needs of nursing guidance for self-care of clients on hemodialysis therapy. *Rev Bras Enferm* 2011; 64: 335-342.
3. Wright Nunes JA. Education of patients with chronic kidney disease at the interface of primary care providers and nephrologists. *Adv Chronic Kidney Dis* 2013; 20: 370-378.
4. Huang X, Carrero JJ. Better prevention than cure: optimal patient preparation for renal replacement therapy. *Kidney Int* 2014; 85: 507-510.

E-mail: geraldobezerrajr@unifor.br

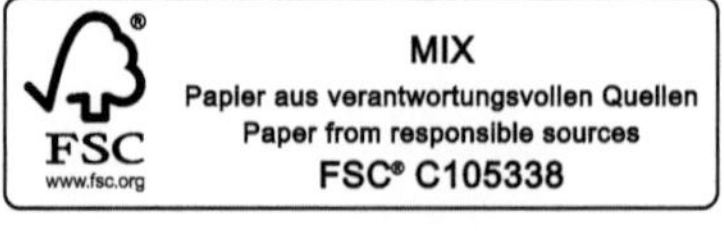

Printed by Books on Demand GmbH, Norderstedt / Germany